MODELS FOR MENTAL DISORDER
Conceptual Models in Psychiatry

SECOND EDITION

Peter Tyrer
MD FRCP FRCPsych MFPHM
Professor of Community Psychiatry,
St Mary's Hospital Medical School,
London, UK

Derek Steinberg
MB BS MPhil FRCPsych
Consultant Psychiatrist and Director,
Adolescent Unit,
Ticehurst House Hospital, Sussex;
lately Consultant Psychiatrist,
Maudsley and Bethlem Royal Hospital,
London, UK

Illustrated by Derek Steinberg

JOHN WILEY & SONS
Chichester · New York · Brisbane · Toronto · Singapore

1st Edition 1987
2nd Edition 1993
Reprinted July 1994, June 1996

Copyright © 1987, 1993 by John Wiley & Sons Ltd,
        Baffins Lane, Chichester,
        West Sussex PO19 1UD, England
        National   Chichester (0243) 779777
        International   +44 243 779777

Other Wiley Editorial Offices

John Wiley & Sons, Inc., 605 Third Avenue,
New York, NY 10158-0012, USA

Jacaranda Wiley Ltd, 33 Park Road, Milton,
Queensland 4064, Australia

John Wiley & Sons (Canada) Ltd, 22 Worcester Road,
Rexdale, Ontario M9W 1L1, Canada

John Wiley & Sons (SEA) Pte Ltd, 37 Jalan Pemimpin #05-04,
Block B, Union Industrial Building, Singapore 2057

Library of Congress Cataloging-in-Publication Data

Tyrer, Peter J.
    Models for mental disorder : conceptual models in psychiatry /
Peter Tyrer, Derek Steinberg ; illustrated by Derek Steinberg. –
2nd ed.
      p. cm.
    Includes bibliographical references and index.
    ISBN 0 471 93983 8
    1. Psychology, Pathological – Philosophy.   I. Steinberg, Derek.
II. Title.
    [DNLM: 1. Mental Disorders.   2. Models, Biological.   3. Models,
Psychological.   WM 100 T992m 1993]
RC437.5.T95   1993
616.89 – dc20
DNLM/DLC
for Library of Congress   93–19006
                                           CIP

British Library Cataloguing in Publication Data

A catalogue record for this book is available from the British Library

ISBN 0 471 93983 8

Typeset in 10/11pt Palatino by Inforum, Rowlands Castle, Hants
Printed and bound in Great Britain by
Biddles Ltd, Guildford and King's Lynn

Contents

Preface To The First Edition

Psychiatry is not yet an exact science. It accommodates a range of disciplines from sociology to biochemistry which approach the subject from different standpoints. As a consequence, confusion often reigns and it is difficult for the uninitiated to know what it is that represents fact, theory and opinion. In order to explain psychiatry it is necessary to use models that offer the practitioner a consistent approach that justifies treatment or investigation. These models are ingenious, clever and convincing but none of them is comprehensive. Nevertheless, they have a major influence on thought and practice and account for a great deal of the debate that goes on in psychiatry.

In this book the main models used in psychiatry are described in straightforward language. They are the biological (disease), psychodynamic, social and behavioural models. Each model serves as its own advocate, presents its credentials and defends itself against the criticisms of other models. The reader can then decide whether or not this is done successfully. In the final chapter an integrated model, termed the correlative model, shows how each approach can be used at different times in the course of a psychiatric illness. The aim is both to clarify the thinking of professionals in psychiatry and explain to the student in social work, psychology and medicine, how conflict and confusion have arisen because protagonists have been arguing from the standpoint of different models. This should prove helpful both in understanding psychiatry and in stimulating thought about a subject which still depends too much on untested theory and opinon.

It is not meant to be a textbook although key references are given at the end of each chapter. Although the jargon of psychiatry is used it is always explained beforehand and the reasons for differences in terminology become clear. The illustrations are intended to clarify and emphasize the text, and may sometimes amuse. After grasping the essential features of each model the student should be able to recognize quickly which model is being used by mental health professionals. Most like to regard themselves as eclectic in that they borrow from each model when it is appropriate but, in truth, few are entirely unbiased in their approach. Our book will help the student to realize that rigid adherence to one of the standard models leads to a blinkered view of mental disorder that hinders the multidisciplinary approach that is such an important part of good practice. Lastly, we trust that after reading this book the student will be stimulated to engage both colleagues and teachers in lively debate, to challenge them when models are used unwisely and to make better sense of a medical discipline that is more often known for its confusion than its clarity.

Peter J Tyrer
Derek Steinberg
December 1986

Preface To The Second Edition

To acknowledge the changes that have taken place in psychiatry in the past few years we have updated all the chapters and also introduced a chapter illustrating the cognitive model. In revising the main models we have caricaturized them to a lesser extent than in the first edition, although not with any intention to blunt the legitimate criticisms that can be made of them.

We are pleased to note that there is now much less rigidity in applying models in psychiatry than when this book was first planned but the need to explain each of them consistently is still present. We hope our readers are satisfied with the changes in this second edition so that the task of explaining the many facets of psychiatry becomes a more coherent one.

Peter J Tyrer
Derek Steinberg
November 1992

Acknowledgements

We should like to thank our many colleagues for stimulating our interest in model-building and contributing to an integration of them, and especially to John Williams for advice on the behavioural model, Kate Davidson for comments on the cognitive model, Patrick West for encouragement, and to Hazel Hills, Anna Carver, Marlene Whitaker and Sandra Jones for secretarial help in converting our views and occasional ramblings to the printed page.

PT
DS

CHAPTER 1

Introduction

The public image of psychiatry is not an attractive one. It is not a single image but more a set of incompatible impressions, of earnest bearded men with Germanic accents hovering over recumbent clients, of impersonal white-coated figures in spotless clinics administering drugs and similar treatments to patients with barely a word of communication, of wild and woolly therapists talking incomprehensively about protest and despair, and of cosy reassuring figures delivering common sense whilst pretending it is derived from the methods of science. All these images are caricatures. It is as though the public were looking at psychiatry in a gallery of distorting mirrors, each mirror emphasizing one aspect of the subject at the expense of the rest, and yet all appearing equally grotesque.

With this mixture of impressions it is hardly surprising that the subject appears irrational and confused. Unfortunately this impression is justified and cannot just be blamed on public relations. There is no indication that psychiatry has a common theoretical base and each practitioner seems to have an idiosyncratic approach which is often at complete variance from that of his colleagues. It is often said that if you want five different opinions on any aspect of mental health you just need to ask five psychiatrists. If each opinion is contradictory the impression of incompetence and inadequacy is given to the discipline and its practitioners.

As an example of how confusion can arise let us look at a common problem in psychiatric practice, a person who develops persistent depression following the death of a close relative. This can be perceived in several ways by psychiatrists. One sees the depression as a pathological event that is directly due to the biochemical change occurring in the brain of someone who is predisposed to

1

pathological depression through an accident of heredity, as it is known that there is a genetic component in depressive illness. Another sees the depression as a reactivation of unresolved childhood conflicts over an early loss. Another regards the depression as part of the normal mourning process that has got out of control because the person's thoughts become fixed in a negative set which sees everything in the most pessimistic light. Yet others conclude that the mourning response has been exaggerated primarily by society, or see it as an abnormal form of learning which is no longer appropriate for the situation but is receiving encouragement from some quarter (positive reinforcement). It is easy to see that these contradictory views about the cause of the psychiatric problem become even more magnified when one considers the course of the illness, its treatment, and prevention of recurrence.

The reader may well be aware of these strong differences of opinion but they tend to be minimized in many texts on mental illness. The textbook author's aim is to present a clear and concise account of the subject which is internally logical and consistent yet reflects the subject as a whole. At present this is almost impossible to achieve in psychiatry; the only way to be clear, simple and logical is to present a biased view that can only be consistent by selective omission of alternative views. When other approaches and attitudes are mentioned they stand out by their strangeness and provoke questions that cannot be answered satisfactorily.

In practice conflict is predictable and increases proportionately with the number of psychiatrists and related professionals involved with a particular problem. The reason for the conflict is not that psychiatrists are necessarily ignorant, ill-trained or confused or woolly thinkers by nature, but that psychiatry as a discipline is still immature. Knowledge in psychiatry is far outstripped by theories and opinions and these are allowed to flourish because the evidence needed to contradict them is not available.

When faced with limited information people use models in an attempt to create order and cohesion from their subject. A model can either explain a set of facts or views and thereby increase understanding, or represent a goal that should be the aim of a particular course of action.

It is interesting that in normal usage the word model has two meanings, one of explanation and the other of imitation, that are essentially similar. The best model satisfies both requirements and does so with the least distortion of known facts. Of course one can take the view that facts in science are not true in the absolute sense but are only the best available approximation to the truth at present (Popper 1963) and so a model may be correct even if it fails to fit the

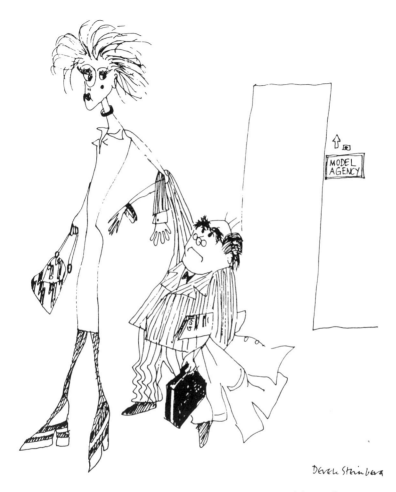

'Models cause psychiatrists endless trouble . . .'

facts. In these cases the word only satisfies one of its definitions and is best regarded as a hypothesis rather than a model. Models are essentially practical instruments that follow existing knowledge rather than break new ground. Although Engel (1977) has stated that 'a model is nothing more than a belief system' many beliefs are quite at variance with existing knowledge and are no use as models. For example, there is a model of mental illness that states that all mental disorder is the will of God and is a punishment for our sins. A large number of people still believe this model but the available evidence does not suggest that saints are free from psychiatric disturbance or that major sinners have more mental illness than minor sinners. The more a model has to rely on belief rather than factual evidence the less appropriate it will be. Models cause psychiatrists endless trouble and we should like to do without them but this can only happen when the subject explains itself so well that further simplification is redundant.

We all like to have a coherent basis for our actions and psychiatrists are no exception. Most psychiatrists, usually implicitly, adopt one of the psychiatric models we shall be discussing. Explicitly they may claim that they come to a considered judgement on each issue and adopt the appropriate model for that judgement. They thus regard themselves as eclectic but although this sounds impressive it describes neither a model nor a philosophy. In practice the eclectic follows his own admitted or undeclared prejudices and then cannot understand why all his colleagues do not agree with him. It allows the luxury of change without giving a reason and is not far short of pure empiricism, a philosophy that states that everything should be based on experience.

None of the models of mental illness we shall describe is a paragon of elegance. They cannot deal with all the material of psychiatry neatly and crisply, leaving no loose ends. It is because of this that model-making attracts such interest in psychiatry; the search is on for a model which is truly comprehensive and can be applied universally. In other branches of medicine the theoretical framework for the doctor's actions is better established, so looking for new models is less urgent. The cause, clinical manifestations, pathology and treatment of much organic illness is known and the disease model, the details of which we shall come across later, is admirably suited to the subject matter. Unfortunately, as we shall find, the disease model often fails us in psychiatry and stretching it to encompass all mental disorder is a Procrustean exercise.

Rather than present a cosmetic repair of the schisms in psychiatric thought, we think that the divisions should be exposed from the beginning. In the following chapters we leave each model to speak for itself in explaining the cause and pathology of, and selecting the right treatment for, a number of psychiatric problems. Examples are then described in the form of case histories. Each case is interpreted using the model under consideration, highlighting the advantages and disadvantages of each model in practice. By doing this the differences between the models are emphasized and only in the final chapter do we try and reconcile them. We hope that by exposing the conflict between the models the reason for the confusion in the subject becomes clear, and that there can be greater understanding, of the psychiatrist's attempts to give convincing explanations for his actions. It should also help the reader to decide which are the important components of mental illness, a decision which will obviously depend on the model with which he is most at home. We do not pretend that our synthesis in the final chapter is going to satisfy all criticisms but at least it offers a framework for use in practice that can be described as reasonably comprehensive. At present there is room for all models, but in time a unifying approach should come. In the meantime it is essential to expose all the models to scrutiny, accepting their deficiencies as well as their advantages.

It will surprise no-one that there is argument over the number of models used in psychiatry and how they should be classified. Siegler & Osmond (1974), in their comprehensive account of models in psychiatry, describe six; medical, moral, psychoanalytic, family, conspiratorial and social. We have confined our attention to four; the disease model, which is often confused with the so-called medical model, a term that we reject with Bursten (1979) as a rhetorical device that obscures more than it clarifies, the psychodynamic, behavioural (roughly equivalent to Siegler & Osmond's use of moral) and social models. We feel that these four models can be examined separately because each can stand alone in explaining the cause and course of psychiatric illness, its management and prevention.

This is not intended to be a short textbook of psychiatry. Much of the time we shall be talking about ideas, views and opinions, and these are no substitute for the bricks and mortar of hard fact. Nevertheless, our aim is the practical one of making sense of psychiatry, so we do not confuse with a mass of contradictory information. At its simplest level we are trying to teach a simple sorting operation, like the tests often given to young children in which they are required to separate a number of articles on the basis of shape, size or colour. If this book is to serve its purpose you should be able quickly to identify each new piece of psychiatric information and place it with the appropriate model. There should be little difficulty in identifying the right model for a particular item as there is relatively little overlap between them. This applies to all types of information, whether or not couched in the language of psychiatric jargon. So Lady Macbeth's question, 'Canst thou not minister to a mind diseased, pluck from the heart a rooted sorrow?' can be quickly tagged with the psychodynamic label, as it both recognizes a personal illness and suggests a psychotherapeutic technique in correcting it. This view receives confirmation later in the play when Lady Macbeth explains 'Throw physic to the dogs, I'll none of it', as a rejection of one model by the adherents of another is a well-recognized phenomenon.

Of course the sorting process is only the first stage in using models properly, but if it is done wrongly it will be impossible to build up an internally logical system which incorporates all the information. Once we have these internal systems, learning becomes a great deal easier. What originally appears to be a pot-pourri of isolated facts and opinions becomes not only clearer but also more interesting when it makes sense. Because treatment is closely linked to each model the disturbingly large range of therapies in psychiatry falls into perspective. The final enterprise is the synthesis of the models, a synthesis which we have attempted but realize its limitations. To some extent each practitioner has to make a personal synthesis, an exercise which demands a great deal but amply repays in results. We are not expecting all who read this book to get to the stage of personal model building but hope at least that any views that are already held are recognized as components of a model rather than visitations of truth. Both an honest self-assessment and understanding of the curious ways in which psychiatry is practised are the first steps in recognizing the subject as it really is. This is important for existing psychiatrists to understand each other, for students and aspiring psychiatrists to understand their teachers, and for all of us, in our capacity as potential patients, to understand the thinking of our therapists.

REFERENCES

Bursten, B. (1979) Psychiatry and the rhetoric of models. *American Journal of Psychiatry*, **136**, 661–665.

Engel, G.L. (1977) The need for a new medical model: a challenge for medicine. *Science*, **196**, 129–136.

Popper, K. (1963) *Conjecture and Refutations: the Growth of Scientific Knowledge*. Routledge and Kegan Paul, London.

Siegler, M. and Osmond, H. (1974) *Models of Madness: Models of Medicine*. MacMillan, New York.

CHAPTER 2

The Disease Model

'The main claim of the physical approach, that is the assumption that mental disorders are dependent on physiological changes, is that it is a useful working hypothesis. It has made great advances and looks like making more. It is in line with the main front of biological advance. It is here where psychiatry belongs.'

Eliot Slater, 1954

The name 'mental illness' implies disease. An illness suggests there is something wrong that is fundamentally different from normal function and is not just a variation in degree. The disease model regards mental malfunction as a consequence of physical and chemical changes primarily in the brain but sometimes in other parts of the body. It is a model that has served general medicine extremely well over the last millenium, and particularly so in the past 200 years. It implies that in mental illness there is a considerable degree of impaired function and pathological change, and that such illness can be regarded as disease. The definition of disease is not an easy task but has to be faced by the model. The central components of a disease are its qualitative difference from normal variation and its conferment of handicap on the individual. Scadding (1967) defines disease as 'the sum of the abnormal phenomena displayed by a group of living organisms in association with a specified common characteristic or set of characteristics by which they differ from the norm for their species in such a way as to place them at a biological disadvantage'. This definition is equally suited to physical and psychiatric disease and is important because it sets limits to illness. In psychiatry for example, disorders of personality are often considered to be psychiatric illnesses, but are not necessarily biologically disadvantageous and

7

merge imperceptibly into normal variation (e.g. suicide, homicide, being murdered, child abuse, etc.). The disease model of psychiatry considers many of these conditions to be beyond its scope and unsuitable for psychiatric treatment.

There are basically four stages of illness that are described by the disease model, but at times these may be extended to six. The exact nature of each of these stages may take many years to elucidate fully and our knowledge of many illnesses remains incomplete because the elucidation of pathology is so difficult. Frequently the answer to the critical question that apparently should explain everything only begs another question that had not previously been considered. Our knowledge of almost all mental illness is incomplete because one or more of these stages remains a mystery, but this should not mean that the disease model should be abandoned. Once all the stages are recognized the illness belongs firmly in the province of medicine and can be treated predictably and consistently. The stages tend to be determined chronologically and are (1) the description of the symptoms and main features of the disorder (the clinical syndrome), (2) identification of pathology (i.e. the structural or biochemical changes caused by illness), (3) close study of the natural history of the syndrome, and (4) determining its cause or causes. Management or treatment based on the pathology of the illness and the outcome following that treatment (prognosis) can also be considered as part of the model, but if all the other stages are determined these will follow automatically.

DESCRIPTION OF THE CLINICAL SYNDROME

Almost invariably the recognition of a clinical syndrome is the first stage in the identification of an illness. This begins by noting that certain symptoms such as loss of appetite and lack of energy, or objective signs such as a rapid pulse and an enlarged thyroid gland, tend to be associated in certain illnesses. Once the investigator's mind is alerted to this link other symptoms or signs are identified until the complete syndrome is found. The persistent association of two symptoms or signs may be a chance finding, three is likely to imply a real association, and four confirms it. Observation is the hallmark of correct identification of the syndrome and depends on clinical skills alone. The different elements of the syndrome may have no obvious meaning at first but they will all have to be accounted for if a syndrome is to achieve the status of a disease. Doctors such as Sydenham and Bright in the 18th century were excellent examples of syndrome detectors, and unlike modern doctors they did not have the technology of the laboratory to help them in their task. The great fictional detective, Sherlock Holmes, was modelled on the clinical skills of a well-known Scottish physician, Sir Charles Bell, who was famed for his ability to diagnose medical conditions from small tell-tale signs that no-one else had noticed.

Through clinical observation alone such doctors identified forms of disease which were only shown to have the other attributes of the disease model many years later. For example, acute Bright's disease is an inflammation of the kidney (nephritis), first described 150 years ago. Bright suspected that the syndrome of fever, swelling of the face and hands and little or no flow of urine (anuria) was likely to involve the kidney, but until he linked all the clinical symptoms together the illness went unrecognized. It was many years later before the microscopic pathology (an inflammation of certain structures (glomeruli) of the kidney) and the cause (hypersensitivity to certain strains of a bacterium (the haemolytic streptococcus)) were discovered, but it was Bright who first focused the eyes of science on the problem.

Clinical syndromes are later refined into diagnoses, which are really convenient code names for the syndromes. So when doctors talk together about a patient with thyrotoxicosis (Graves' disease) they are telling each other in one word that the patient has a syndrome which is likely to include an enlarged thyroid gland (goitre) together with atypical facial appearance, loss of weight, abnormal trembling, special eye signs, rapid heartbeat, increased speed of reflexes and nervousness. The diagnosis of an illness may not be confirmed until other tests (usually carried out in a laboratory) are also consistent with the disease in question but it is accepted that the important part of the diagnostic process is the clinical assessment of the patient, and a clinical diagnosis can stand independently of laboratory findings.

The assessment consists of a detailed history from the patient and a careful physical examination. The history gives strong clues about the possible nature of the complaint, so that the doctor is sensitized to pay special attention to certain features when he carries out his examination. Because a history can be unreliable or may omit important changes he should always carry out a full physical examination, for even if he finds an abnormality expected from the history he might miss other abnormal signs unless all systems are examined.

Every medical student learns this basic approach at an early stage in training and it is also expected by the general public. 'He didn't even examine me' is a common complaint among patients who visit their doctor and are not satisfied by the reassurance or treatment given after a six-minute consultation (the average duration of consultations in general practice). Psychiatrists who follow the disease model have a very similar approach to the assessment of mental symptoms. The first stage is a careful history which is more detailed and usually takes longer than a medical history. This is because the background of the patient, his personal and family history, and his personality are assessed as well as any relevant medical and psychiatric history. All psychiatrists, whatever model they adopt, have to take the whole man into account in making an assessment. Every doctor pays lip-service to this holistic approach but may ignore it in practice as the knowledge derived may not affect treatment significantly. If a patient consults a doctor for removal of a wart (verruca) on his finger he would take exception to a full exposé of his personal and sexual life on the grounds that this information was irrelevant to wart removal. The psychiatrist who follows the disease model is sometimes criticized for not thinking of the patient as a person, but as a 'case'. The criticism, which is common in other branches of medicine, is only justified if the doctor treats the problem wrongly because of inadequate assessment. But even if a psychiatrist looks on a mental disorder as a brain disease he cannot afford to neglect a full history of past and present problems as this gives important clues to the nature of the disorder. Where he will differ from his colleagues who follow different models is that his questions will be more formalized and the interactional part of the interview ingored. The interview is regarded as an exercise to gain information instead of the first phase in a personal relationship.

The physical examination is carried out in the same way as in other medical conditions, and is an essential part of the assessment of every psychiatric patient, even though it may provide no additional information, as only a few psychiatric disorders have obviously abnormal physical signs. Some psychiatrists disregard a physical examination on the grounds that they are only specialists in mental health, and feel that psychologists and social workers are just as competent as they are in the assessment of mental health. This annoys the disease psychiatrist. The late Dr Richard Hunter, one of the strongest adherents to the disease model, attacks this view in trenchant terms, 'Psychiatrists do not diagnose their patients like other doctors do. They discard four of their senses and literally play it by ear.

It is the no-touch technique adapted to new purpose. Physical examination or laboratory investigation, which transformed medicine from guesswork and theory to fact and science, are spurned or positively discouraged. It is alleged that they deflect attention from study in depth of the patient's mind, and impede rapport' (Hunter 1973).

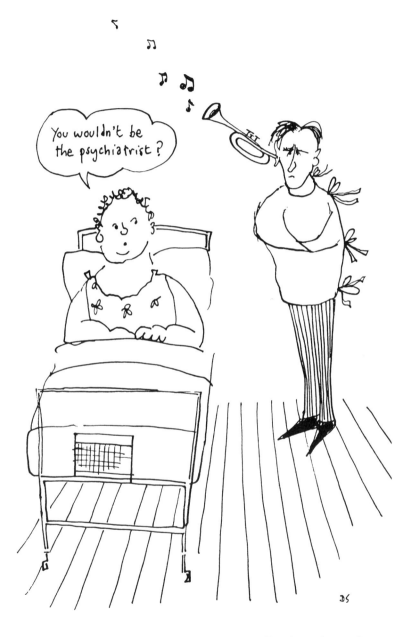

'They discard four of their senses and literally play it by ear'

The same principles apply when carrying out an examination of the mental state. Although laboratory and other independent tests are not available to confirm the clinical findings the aim remains one of scientific objectivity. The examination of the mental state is the mental equivalent of the physical examination. The psychiatrist already has strong clues from the history to which parts of the mental state are likely to be abnormal but again he must carry out the whole procedure as the history may be unreliable and there may be deliberate attempts to cover up the mental disturbance. The information he gets from the mental state examination is still not entirely objective (the adjectives 'soft' and 'hard' are often used to describe the differences in the quality of data) but it is still very useful and is more reliable than the history.

In the same way that other doctors use a formal jargon to describe abnormal features on examination, such as 'generalized lymphadenopathy' for enlargement of lymph glands throughout the body, psychiatrists use a formal jargon to describe abnormal features in the mental state. This is called descriptive psychopathology or phenomenology, and its development owes a great deal to the work of Karl Jaspers (1963). The interviewer is trying to describe as objectively as possible the abnormal mental features elicited from his examination. By doing so he can summarize the findings in a form which will be informative to others and which otherwise would be an idiosyncratic assessment.

It is not sufficient merely to record the presence of the abnormality but to qualify it in the same way that a doctor will qualify a description such as hepatomegaly (enlarged liver) by saying how many fingerbreadths the liver is enlarged underneath the costal (rib) margin and whether it is hard or soft. For example, the judgement that events going on about you such as people talking amongst themselves and programmes on radio and television refer especially to you, is described in phenomenology as 'ideas of reference', and the feelings of puzzlement and uncertainty that are common in the early stages of schizophrenia, when the patient suspects that something of great significance is happening but which he cannot yet identify, are called 'delusional mood'. The use of such terms greatly simplifies description in psychiatry and experience has shown that patients have a relatively small repertoire of abnormal mental functions in which certain phenomenological elements recur again and again.

The chief disadvantage of the information gathered in this way is that, like the history, it requires the patient's cooperation and depends largely on interpretation of what is said. Although an important part of the mental state examination is observation of the patient during the history and examination, it is rarely sufficient to assess a

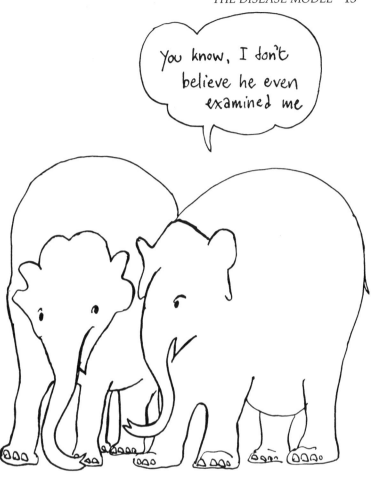

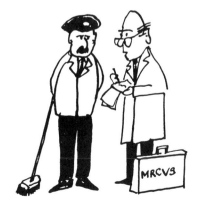

problem alone, so special procedures are necessary for mute and uncooperative patients. Nevertheless, by formalizing the subjective information from the patient the psychiatrist can summarize the disease in a few sentences. He is seldom able to make a diagnosis in a single word as can his medical colleagues, but his equivalent 'diagnostic formulation' is the most economical way he can communicate his findings.

Let us see how this works in practice. First of all we can look at one of the most common mental symptoms, depression, but it is useful to take as an example a condition that is relatively rare but which satisfies all the stages of the disease model. The format of the history and examination is the same for all psychiatric assessments employing the disease model and is shown in ordinary type. The interpretation of the information according to the model is shown in italics.

STAGE 1 CASE HISTORY—DESCRIPTION OF CLINICAL SYNDROME

History

The patient is a young man of 24, referred to an outpatient clinic after a referral from the general practitioner. In the general practitioner's referal letter the essential elements are contained in two sentences. 'He has become much more withdrawn, and both his family and I think his personality has changed. He is much more suspicious of people and does not trust anybody; he does not trust me now because he has come repeatedly with complaints about his health and is not satisfied that I can find nothing physically wrong.'

Main complaint: 'You can't help me. I need the police. Those people outside want to kill me and they're taking over my mind as well.' *Delusions suspected, particularly paranoid ones and those of mind control (passivity).*

Family history: Father 54, an inventor. Has only had one major success, a patented can-opener, and has lived on the income from this for much of his life. Has always been an isolated man with few friends; preoccupied with pollution and healthy food. Has never trusted other people. Had one occasion in the past when he felt the landlord was trying to harass him into leaving a rented property and his general practitioner asked for a psychiatric opinion. He would not accept treatment and compulsory admission to hospital was considered inappropriate. Since then has been suspicious of general practitioners and rarely consults them. *Father is likely to have a paranoid personality disorder and may have had a paranoid psychotic episode in the past.* Mother, 50, divorced from husband five years ago. Quick-tempered, gregarious, never able to adjust to husband's self-imposed isolation and paranoia and left him for another man.

Patient an only child. Apart from father, a paternal uncle suffered from a mental illness thought to be schizophrenia. He had many admissions to hospital and committed suicide by jumping from a 10-storey building at the age of 49. *Both father and uncle appear to have had schizophrenia or schizophreniform (schizophrenia-like) illnesses. This may be relevant to the patient's own condition as schizophrenia is transmitted partly by genetic factors.*

Personal history: Born in an industrial town in the south of England. No birth problems, early development difficulties or childhood illnesses apart from measles. *No physical problems present in early life which might predispose him to psychiatric disorder.* Local primary and secondary schools, no special abilities, left at 16. Worked as a bookshop assistant for five years but eventually was sacked because of poor time-keeping. Said he had lost interest in this work and could not be bothered to keep to the times of normal working. Has not tried to get a job since but feels he has special abilities as a thinker and the Government might ask him to work for them at some point in the future because of these abilities. Lives with father. Little contact with him, but he regards this as satisfactory and does not want to have a closer relationship. Has no close friends and little contact with women. 'I've never had a girlfriend, I've just had occasional sexual relationships with prostitutes.' Has no wish to get married or have any closer relationships with women.

Previous personality: Has always been a 'loner'. Regards other people as potentially threatening and finds it best to stay away from them. Used to collect stamps; no longer does so but regards his collection as special, and regards it as more important than any of his personal relationships. *The patient shows definite evidence of a schizoid personality disorder as described in the tenth revision of the International Classification of Disease (ICD-10) (World Health Organisation, 1992). The combination of eccentricity, lack of emotional warmth and confiding relationships, and a preference for solitary activities are all typical features of this personality type.*

History of present condition: Over the past two years he has become increasingly concerned that people have been trying to harm him.

When asked to explain this he said that the problems all began when the traffic lights at the crossroads outside his house ceased to work for a few days. Almost immediately afterwards he developed the notion that other people were following him and came to the conclusion that the traffic light failure was a deliberate signal to 'these people'. He claimed that he could recognize these people because they communicated by a technique which involved jangling their loose change inside their pockets. The young man therefore was able to detect these people when they were standing in bus queues or standing in the street. In the past six months he claimed these people were communicating with him in special ways. 'They can read my mind. They are aliens from another planet. They want to kill me so that they can take over my body in the same way they have taken over the bodies of all the other people who are following me. They won't be satisfied until they have taken me over com-pletely.' *History indicates paranoid delusions and auditory hallucinations.*

Physical Examination

Tall, thin man, weighing 69 kg, 1.8 m tall. No abnormalities noted on physical examination.

Mental state examination: Extremely suspicious during interview, looking furtively about the room and on one occasion become very agitated when he thought he heard someone jangling change inside his pockets in the corridor. His talk was intense and hesitant as though he was afraid of being overheard. He frequently talked irrel-evantly and some of his speech was difficult to follow (e.g. 'I know they can read my mind. Did you hear that noise? That tells me they are reading it now. I know I have the answer. The lights are off; they must go on again. They can kill me now if they want. I have my sword but I will not defend myself'). *Shows thought disorder typical of schizophrenia with lack of obvious connection between sentences.* He was convinced that aliens were controlling his mind as they could both pick up his thoughts and make him think what they wanted him to think. 'I can be part of them. They know my mind; they are in my mind. I must do exactly what they say. They are in control.' *Shows the phenomenon of 'passivity' together with gross thought disorder (in-cluding thought broadcasting and thought control with thought insertion). The belief that his mind is an empty vessel which is controlled by an alien force and that there is nothing he can do about it is one of the characteristic features of schizophrenia.* Can hear the voices of people he regards as aliens talking to him, telling him to do things, and also talking about him among themselves. They say things like 'he's not doing what we want; he must be half asleep. We'll have to wake him up'. Believes the voices come from space or possibly from another planet. He has never seen the aliens. *Has auditory hallucinations (i.e. the perception of hearing voices without the obvious stimulus of the voice). Some of these voices describe him in the third person and this too is typical of schizophrenia.*

On testing his memory, he is able to remember a name and address after five-minute recall and to do simple calculations like subtracting seven from a hundred and subsequent subtractions of seven from the number produced. Is up to date with world affairs but not with local ones. Knows the date, time and place of interview. *He shows no significant intellectual impairment and is orientated in time and space.*

After this structured interview a diagnostic formulation is constructed. This summarizes the nature of the abnormal mental state and suggests a plan of management which will both determine the final diagnosis and appropriate treatment. In this case the formulation could read 'a young man with an apparent schizoid personality disorder who has become excessively suspicious, with auditory hallucinations and thought disorder, believing that his mind is being controlled by aliens. These symptoms are experienced in a clear consciousness and the provisional diagnosis is that of paranoid schizophrenia (ICD-10 – Code 20.0).

Although the diagnosis may appear clear at this stage there are several other conditions that could give rise to a similar clinical picture, including the abuse of drugs such as amphetamines and LSD, or, more rarely, physical disease such as temporal lobe epilepsy. These conditions will have to be excluded before the diagnosis of paranoid schizophrenia is made definitely.

The reader will note from this history and assessment that each element is interpreted, mainly in the shorthand of psychiatric description to aid communication, and that the assessment concentrates on those phenomena that are demonstrated, not those which are hidden or unconscious.

STAGE 2—IDENTIFICATION OF PATHOLOGY

Clinical medicine cannot be practised well without other independent evidence that either confirms or refutes the diagnostic hints derived from clinical examination. The science of pathology is an essential handmaiden to good practice, and a range of investigations from simple estimations of haemoglobin concentration, electrolytes and liver function tests (from blood), to more complex tests such as computer assisted tomography (CAT) scans of different parts of the body, and examination of tissues obtained by biopsy or surgical removal, all help to hone the diagnosis, select treatment and predict prognosis.

In mental illness this is more difficult, because most mental disorder is not accompanied by obvious physical pathology. It is the demonstration of the specific features of schizophrenia described in the previous section, particularly the phenomenon of passivity, that replaces laboratory tests and helps to clinch the diagnosis of schizophrenia. Of course this is not without risk; patients may simulate the diagnostic features of a disorder, or may only have them for such a short time that they do not qualify for schizophrenic diagnosis, but this is no reason to decry them. It is remarkable that the symptoms of schizophrenia are virtually the same in all cultures and all races; people are not the same but illnesses are.

Laboratory and other investigations to determine pathology may still help, and in the case of the young man described above, were helpful in confirming that he had not taken drugs of abuse (by a urine screen), that he had no abnormalities of white or red blood cells, and no electrolyte disturbance. A CAT or NMR (nuclear magnetic resonance) scan might also have been considered, because there is evidence of abnormalities in the temporal lobes of some schizophrenic patients that are demonstrated by outlining the ventricles of the brain and indicating selective dilatation (Bebbington and McGuffin 1988). However, the clinical value of this information is not yet clear and such investigations are not routine, although before long they are likely to be.

Mental symptoms may also be the precursors of physical disease and are therefore more sensitive detectors than more conventional tests. Von Economo's disease, for example, is a form of encephalitis that was first described in 1917 and became an epidemic in the 1920s before apparently dying out. Tiredness and extreme withdrawal (stupor) alternated with confusion and excitement in the acute phase and and there was often nothing abnormal found on physical examination. The later development of the disorder occurred many years later after apparent return to normality following the acute illness. The disease associated with reduced functioning in the parts of the brain concerned with coordinating movement and posture (Parkinson's disease) emerged 20 years or more after the original episode. It would be easy to regard these two phases as separate illnesses but they are part of the same disease process. The mental symptoms may be an important clue to the presence of a disease and it is up to the doctor to describe them accurately and intimately rather than dismiss them as psychological detritus.

STAGE 3—NATURAL HISTORY OF THE SYNDROME

By taking the natural history of a disease (i.e. its course from beginning to end in the absence of treatment) into account, it is possible to improve the sensitivity of diagnosis. Thus it is now established that some people develop some (usually), or all (occasionally) of the symptoms of schizophrenia for very short periods only. Such illnesses are now called 'schizophreniform' (i.e. have the appearance of schizophrenia without necessarily being schizophrenia). Thus to acquire the diagnosis of paranoid schizophrenia in ICD-10 it is necessary for the symptoms to 'have been clearly present for most of the time during a period of one month or more' (World Health Organisation 1992). For those with shorter episodes other diagnoses are available, but these may be revised subsequently to paranoid schizophrenia after the passage of time and with increased information.

Of course the natural history may be an intermittent or irregular one with no obvious pattern. But even here there can be important clues from the history. There is another rare but important disease, acute intermittent porphyria, which presents as severe attacks of abdominal pain and confusion. These attacks may be provoked by certain drugs such as barbiturates. So if a patient awaiting an operation in hospital is given a barbiturate to aid sleep the night before the operation, an attack of porphyria can be triggered. As the disease is rare it is frequently undetected at first, and mental illness labels such as 'hysteria' are frequently applied to the attacks. In time, however, the pattern of the attacks should give the clue to the diagnosis.

STAGE 4—MATCHING DIAGNOSIS TO TREATMENT

Genetic studies of the disease are necessary to establish the relative importance of environmental and constitutional factors in the causation of illness, and even if there is no evidence of an environmental cause the disorder may still be due to an illness that is transmitted by hereditary factors. This has been shown with both schizophrenia and manic depressive (affective) psychoses, in which the standard technique of the geneticist, the study of the disease in monozygotic or identical (derived from a single cell) and dizygotic or nonidentical (derived from two separate cells) twins, reared together or apart, has revealed a high genetic loading. If the illness is hereditary, there is a greater risk of the second twin developing the illness if the first twin has the disorder in monozygotic compared with dizygotic twins. As the monozygotic twin has exactly the same genes as his co-twin this higher rate can only be explained by the disease having a hereditary basis.

Once all these stages of the disease model have been established, treatment often follows without any further knowledge being necessary, as in our young man with schizophrenia. But as we have found already, all too few of the mental illnesses we come across can be analysed in this comprehensive way. In the incomplete cases the doctor using the disease model adopts the empirical approach. He gives the most effective treatment known for the clinical syndrome he has identified if he knows that its natural history follows a chronic course or he may do nothing if he knows that the condition has a good outcome. He will determine which treatments are most effective through the means of the controlled clinical trial. Clinical trials are often criticized by those who disapprove of the disease model in psychiatry because they allegedly reduce a person to the status of a 'case', and because personal aspects of treatment are removed. Criticism is also made because the controlled clinical trial is an experiment and this is incompatible with treating the whole man. In fact, most of the controlled aspects of a clinical trial involve keeping all but one of the factors affecting outcome as constant as possible so that changes that take place are likely to be a consequence of the only variable not kept constant, the treatments being tested.

In this way conclusions can be made about the effectiveness of the treatment much more rapidly than knowledge gained by trial and error. The demonstration of an effective treatment may also help to discover some of the other stages in the disease model. For example, it is known that most patients with the clinical syndrome of schizophrenia are dramatically improved by treatment with one or more of the antipsychotic group of drugs (major tranquillizers) and will relapse if these drugs are withdrawn (Hirsch *et al.*, 1973). The symptoms of schizophrenia are suppressed and yet other aspects of brain function are unchanged. This, according to the disease model, is evidence of a specific brain abnormality in schizophrenia, which is corrected by drug treatment.

It has recently been confirmed that major tranquillizers are effective in schizophrenia because they block the effects of a naturally occurring amine, dopamine, on certain sites (receptors) in the brain (Johnstone *et al.* 1978). There is also evidence that patients with schizophrenia have a structural abnormality in the brain (temporal lobe) which differentiates them from those with other mental disorders (Brown *et al.* 1986). If this is confirmed the second stage of the disease model, identification of pathology, will soon be complete. The demonstration of an effective treatment would then be seen as a signpost towards discovery of the nature of the illness.

There is abundant evidence in medicine of treatments that were shown to be effective long before it was known how they worked—and with these precedents the disease psychiatrist should have no qualms in defending the empirical approach. So the fuss that some people make over the use of electroconvulsive therapy (ECT) will not trouble him, for he is satisfied by the evidence of clinical trials that for some psychiatric conditions, particularly depressive psychosis (the diagnosis is important), ECT is a highly effective form of treatment and may be life-saving in someone with strong suicidal feelings associated with depression. The fact that a somewhat unusual form of treatment such as ECT is still given without knowing why it works is important for the scientist to elucidate but should not inhibit the therapist from giving it when its effectiveness has been demonstrated (Gregory *et al.* 1985).

The critic may respond by claiming that the disease model is unjustified in assuming that all the psychiatric conditions over which it claims authority are diseases in the accepted sense. It is not good enough to presume that in time a bodily pathology will be found in such conditions as depression and schizophrenia. The demonstration of pathology should precede therapeutic intervention, particularly for those procedures such as prefrontal leucotomy, in which treatment is irreversible. This criticism can be countered on empirical grounds—if we waited until we were certain what was wrong before starting treatment most of current therapy would have to cease forthwith—but it also brings up the question of the dividing line between disease and non-disease in psychiatry. This is not so easy to answer, but most accept Scadding's view (1967) that to qualify for a disease label a medical condition must be biologically disadvantageous. In other words, it must either harm the individual or reduce his or her capacity to reproduce.

Taking this as the criterion for disease several psychiatric conditions can be excluded and the boundary between normality and illness becomes defined. The condition 'hysteria' which is impossible to diagnose except by exclusion of other pathology, is not included as formal mental illness. The classical symptoms of 'conversion' and 'dissociation' are said by psychodynamic psychiatrists to be unconsciously motivated and secure some advantage for the victim, commonly called 'secondary gain'. Quite apart from the inability to assess unconscious motivation in a formal examination of the mental state, which necessarily implies that no conscious indication of it will be shown to the examiner, the idea that a symptom produces some advantage is incompatible with the disease concept. Hysteria as a diagnosis, therefore, is not permissible. As Slater (1965) concluded, it is 'not only a delusion but also a snare'. There are many psychiatric disorders which grade, apparently imperceptibly, between normality and illness, but the disease model can categorize them adequately. Mental handicap, for example, includes people who are so severely retarded that they are incapable of performing independently the simplest tasks necessary to ensure survival, and also those who can live independently but can only take up simple occupations because of their limited intelligence. The latter would not come into the disease category of mental subnormality; whereas the first group would, according to Scadding's criteria. Probably 'mental handicap' should best be used as a term to describe intellectual functioning, and the term 'disease' involved when there is identifiable brain pathology, as is the case for most people with very severe mental handicap.

There are several other approaches to practice which accompany the disease model. The emphasis on adequate diagnosis and formal classification of psychiatric conditions means that patients are placed in groups and common methods of treatment sought for them. The critic immediately responds by condemning the crudity of a system that regards patients as cases and not as unique individuals who should be dealt with on an individual basis. The disease model's proponents dismiss this as emotive nonsense, arguing that if every patient's condition is regarded as unique in all respects then psychiatry is not a medical discipline but a lottery in which we learn something from each patient but forget it all when we move to the next one. The combination of characteristics that make up a mental disorder is unique, but there are common features that, in a good classification, are found in all other patients within the group, and by using the body of information derived from previous knowledge of the disorder, a more logical and effective system of management can be chosen. As Rutter & Gould (1985) have pointed out in explaining the usefulness of classification in a wider context, it is disorders we are attempting to classify, not people.

Another important facet of the disease model is that the patient is regarded as a passive recipient of treatment. Although the onset and course of the illness is frequently influenced by what the person does, by the time the disease is manifest he is a helpless victim needing external intervention. Just as pneumonia needs antibiotics to reinforce the body's defences against the bacteria that are multi-

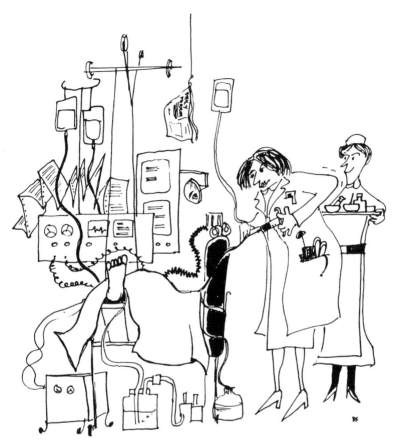

'. . . the patient is regarded as a passive recipient of treatment'

plying rapidly in the lung, the psychiatric patient needs a similar specialist treatment temporarily to replace his normal coping mechanisms. These mechanisms have presumably been employed at an earlier stage in the illness and have demonstrably failed, otherwise the patient would not be seeking specialist advice. Moral exhortations and encouragement are therefore irrelevant to the treatment given according to the disease model. The brain is not functioning properly and the focus of treatment should be directed to the seat of disorder. It is good manners to be considerate to the patient and to respect his rights, and good co-operation means that the patient is more likely to adhere to the treatment prescribed, but it is not an essential part of therapy. The best treatment is the 'magic bullet'—to use the phrase of Paul Ehrlich, one of the first to treat disease scientifically—that eradicates the focus of disease without harming any healthy parts of the body.

As the patient's own part in treatment is relatively small it is not possible to blame failure to respond on the patient on the grounds that he is showing resistance or some other psychodynamic mechanism (a view that is looked on sceptically by those using the disease model as it is incapable of verification). So if a patient with an agreed diagnosis fails to respond to a particular treatment that is normally effective for that illness, then more powerful treatments are selected or the diagnosis is questioned, instead of making the patient responsible for the lack of response. To quote Dr Hunter again 'patients are characterized by epithets which insult their personality and intelligence. Their sufferings are denied by being described in terms of "will not" where body doctors would say "can not" and try to discover why. No other specialty blames illness—and therapeutic failures—on patients'.

It follows naturally that if the patient has a dependent role in the disease model the doctor has an authoritarian one. As the psychiatrist is approached as an expert for advice he accepts this role and acts accordingly. He responds to criticism that he is being patronizing or condescending by saying that the authoritarian role has accompanied good medicine throughout the centuries. If the patient has faith in the doctor and accepts his judgement, treatment will be more effective. It is also argued that most patients prefer their doctor to be an authoritarian, rather than presenting a phoney equality which only makes patients feel uncomfortable.

The authority of the doctor also affects his relationships with other members of the psychiatric team. A definite hierarchy exists, with the doctors taking precedence over other professional workers such as nurses, psychologists, social workers and occupational therapists. This is because the doctors alone have sufficient training both medicine and psychiatry to exercise clinical responsibility. The disease psychiatrist does not take kindly to working in a multi-disciplinary psychiatric team in which all members are alleged experts and insist on the democratic process.

As psychiatric illness often mimics or foreshadows physical illness it is right and proper for the doctor to be the chief decision maker and head of the team. Following assessment he may delegate responsibility to a greater or lesser degree but will always maintain clinical responsibility for the patient.

The need for occasional compulsory admission and treatment is easily defended by the disease model. Psychiatric illness is due to disordered brain function, and as the brain is concerned with higher elements of consciousness such as judgement and insight it is to be

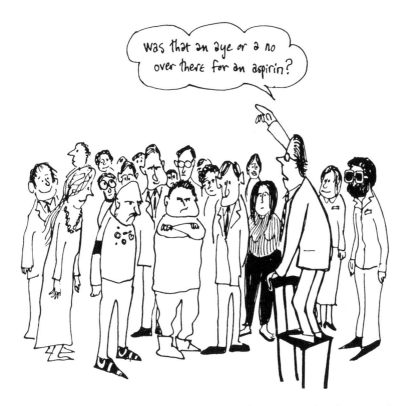

'. . . all members are alleged experts and insist on the democratic process'

expected that often these elements become impaired. If they do, and if the disease can be arrested or cured by treatment, it is appropriate for the doctor to act on behalf of the patient even if it is against the patient's wishes. Just as the first-aid worker does not need consent to practise artificial respiration on the unconscious patient dragged from a swimming pool, the psychiatrist does not necessarily require consent to treat a life-threatening mental illness that has altered the patient's judgement so that he acts and thinks abnormally.

The concept of abnormality is derived from the patient's previous level of functioning before illness and from knowledge of the psychiatric disorder. For example, the so-called manic phase of a manic depressive psychosis is very frequently accompanied by lack of insight. During this phase the patient is overactive and frequently believes himself to be superior to others around him. He can develop grandiose ideas or delusions that he owns a large organization or has supernatural powers. If he is likely to act on these delusions by spending thousands of pounds or attempting to fly from high buildings, admission to hospital is essential. Orders for compulsory admission allow a person's liberty to be taken away if he suffers from an illness that is liable to affect his health adversely or be a danger to others. It is therefore appropriate to treat him against his wishes, knowing from previous experience of this disorder that he will return to his normal self following treatment.

Abnormality according to the disease model is quite different from social abnormality. Compulsory admission is not carried out just because a patient is acting in an antisocial manner. It is true that some illnesses may demonstrate antisocial behaviour as one feature of the disorder but the decision to treat compulsorily is made on the evidence of illness, not on behaviour alone. This is why many psychiatrists will not accept patients as ill just because they are aggressive. If they are acting antisocially and are not ill they should be dealt with by the process of law.

The disease model in psychiatry is presented as a logical and well-tried approach to illnesses of the mind. It is a scientific model and relies on testable theories rather than woolly speculations. As with all science, theories are tested and retested until the best working

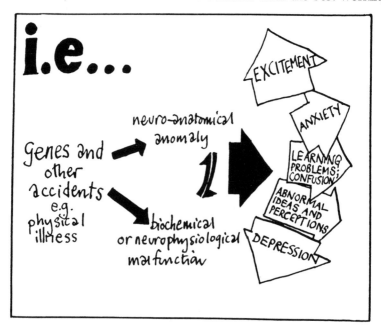

hypothesis is found, only for this to be rejected when it is shown to be inadequate in the light of new knowledge. The model wishes to take away the mythology and mystique from mental illness and replace them with a rational approach that allows psychiatry to come together with other medical disciplines and share in the advances that they have made.

Medical students who read the above account will understand this approach much better than others who are not trained in the same way as doctors. The examination of the patient's mind is similar in many ways to the examination of the body. The main difference is, of course, that we cannot examine the mind physically in the same way we can someone who has a broken leg or a pain in the stomach. You therefore examine the mind indirectly, by analysing some of the most important products of the mind, primarily thoughts expressed in the form of speech. In addition to this the examiner also observes the patient and notes any unusual behaviour in exactly the same way as the doctor examining a patient for a medical illness would observe abnormal physical features such as a mottled complexion, an unusual walk or a skin rash, whether or not it is complained of by the patient. The combination of clinical inquiry eliciting the main psychopathological features together with the keen observation of the detective enables the doctor to come to a diagnosis. This diagnosis is an exact description of a condition which is shared by many other patients and has the great advantage of allowing efficient communication between professionals. A good diagnosis gives an indication of cause, the main clinical features, the recommended treatment and the likely prognosis.

In the case of our patient with suspected paranoid schizophrenia it will be necessary to exclude other causes, including drug abuse (usually quickly done by screening a urine sample for common drugs of abuse), and also exclude other brain disease such as epilepsy. Increasingly brain scans are being used to help with the diagnosis of schizophrenia and in many patients an abnormality is found in the scans because of atrophy (death) of parts of the brain in the hippocampal region. This leads to enlarged ventricles, the spaces between brain matter that are filled with cerebrospinal fluid. Tests such as these are helping to separate schizophrenics into different disorders as it has long been realized that schizophrenia is not a single condition.

DEFENCE OF THE DISEASE MODEL

The practitioner of the disease model is often criticized for failing to see the whole person in his task of identifying a so-called disease in the patient's mind. This criticism is easily dismissed: the good medical doctor does not lose sight of the person when diagnosing hypertension in a 45-year-old bank manager. He has to take notice of this in his recommendations to the person after the high blood pressure has been identified. Advice about work and lifestyle are part of the management of hypertension but the main diagnostic process has to take place independently of this. The doctor has to be satisfied that the high blood pressure is a persistent feature and just not a temporary phenomenon, that it has no immediately treatable cause (i.e. it is essential hypertension), and whether there are particular reasons for not prescribing certain treatments compared with others.

These sort of decisions are clinical ones and exactly the same decisions have to be made by the psychiatrist operating the disease model. Unfortunately the adjective 'clinical' in this setting is often regarded as a rude word. It implies that the psychiatrist has lost his or her humanity, and merely looks at patients as disease objects. When making assessments in a patient with suspected schizophrenia there are no special advantages in being especially sensitive to the person's individuality. Of course each schizophrenic is unique, and so is every case of essential hypertension, but the personal characteristics of the patient should not interfere with the investigation of the disease. The psychiatrist who sends our patient with suspected schizophrenia for an electroencephalogram (EEG) or a neuromagnetic resonance (NMR) scan is not being inhumane or uncaring; he is merely trying to find important treatable causes of the patient's symptoms that might well be forgotten if the main assessment was only of the patient's innermost feelings and how he was reacting to his disorder.

The critic may also reply that whereas diagnoses such as schizophrenia are sometimes appropriate for the disease model, others are quite unsuitable. This criticism is also rebutted. Careful studies show that almost all mental illness, ranging from anxiety following an unpleasant stress to major psychoses such as schizophrenia and manic-depression (affective psychoses), are associated with biochemical, neuropharmacological and hormonal changes. These changes can be measured and are often indicative of pathology. In the broader sense they can therefore be regarded as diseases and the fact that we cannot identify a part of the brain that is pathological at the present state of our knowledge, does not mean that no such change exists. Indeed, schizophrenia was identified at the turn of the century and not found to be associated with any physical disease. It is only in the past 15 years that organic abnormalities have been found with mental patients suffering from this disorder.

Schizophrenia, originally classified as a functional psychosis (i.e. to separate it from organic psychosis in which there was obvious organic pathological change) perhaps should now be classified among the organic ones. The message is clear; it takes many years for the cause and nature of the disease process to be identified in many illnesses. The first step is the identification of the clinical syndrome (using the sensitive diagnostic and observational antennae described above). It is only later, and often much later, that the underlying cause of the syndrome is identified. It is then not unreasonable to think that all mental disorders will in time be shown to be diseases in the medically accepted sense.

REFERENCES

Bebbington, P. and McGuffin, P. (1988) *Schizophrenia: The Major Issues*, Heinemann, London.

Brown, R., Colter, N. *et al.* (1986) Post-mortem evidence of structural brain change in schizophrenia: differences in brain weight, temporal horn area, and para-hippocampal gyrus compared with affective disorder. *Archives of General Psychiatry*, **43**, 36–42.

Goldberger, J., Wheeler, G.A. and Sydenstricker, E. (1918) A study of the diets of non-pellagrous households in textile mill communities in South Carolina. *Journal of the American Medical Association*, **71**, 944–949.

Gregory, S., Shawcross, C.R. and Gill, D. (1985) The Nottingham ECT study: a double-blind comparison of bilateral, unilateral and simulated ECT in depressive illness. *British Journal of Psychiatry*, **146**, 520–524.

Hirsch, S.R., Gaind, R. *et al.* (1973) Outpatient maintenance of chronic schizophrenic patients with long-acting fluphenazine: double-blind placebo trial. *British Medical Journal*, **1**, 633–637.

Hunter, R. (1973) Psychiatry and neurology: psychosyndrome or brain disease? *Journal of the Royal Society of Medicine*, **66**, 359–364.

Jaspers, K. (1963) *General Psychopathology*. Translated by Hoenig, J. and Hamilton, M.W. University Press, Manchester.

Johnstone, E.C., Crow, T.J. *et al.* (1978) Mechanism of the antipsychotic effect in the treatment of acute schizophrenia. *Lancet*, **i**, 848–851.

Popper, K. (1963) *Conjecture and Refutations: the Growth of Scientific Knowledge*. Routledge and Kegan Paul, London.

Rutter, M. and Gould, M. (1985) Classification. In (Rutter, M. and Hersov, L. eds) *Child & Adolescent Psychiatry—Modern Approaches*. Blackwell Scientific Publications, Oxford.

Scadding, J.E. (1967) Diagnosis: the clinician and the computer. *Lancet*, **ii**, 877–882.

Slater, E. (1965) Diagnosis of 'hysteria'. *British Medical Journal*, **1**, 1395–1399.

World Health Organisation (1992) *International Classification of Diseases*, 10th Edn. WHO, Geneva.

CHAPTER 3

The Psychodynamic Model

'There are nine and sixty ways of conducting tribal lays,
And every single one of them is right.'
                    Rudyard Kipling *In The Neolithic Age*

We should begin by explaining that there are many misconceptions about the psychodynamic model, even supposing that a single model can be said to exist; rather it may be better to think of the psychodynamic approach as a particular style of clinical thinking. It follows from this that even among its adherents there is a good deal of argument over the essential elements of the psychodynamic approach, which comprises many quite different conceptions of theory and practice.

The variety of practice that comes broadly into the psychodynamic sphere of influence illustrates that, contrary to what some of its critics say, psychodynamic thinking has not stood still, fossilized, since the late 19th and early 20th century when its basic tenets were being developed by Freud, Jung, Adler and their followers. It has made many significant advances since, but these developments have been in terms of refining concepts, making connections with other disciplines (notably biology and social science), and in new types of clinical practice. It is true that there remain purists who have tended to disown some of the new developments; one of us, attending a conference which sought to show the useful interconnections between biological, social and psychodynamic models, heard a distinguished French psychoanalyst sum up the meeting by thundering that he had learned nothing new or of interest, and that the family therapists (he singled them out) must have had something wrong with their training. Nevertheless we would identify family therapy, group therapy, many aspects of psychotherapy and counselling, much of the creative therapies (e.g. art therapy) and some interesting developments in organizational psychology (i.e. the psychological study of institutions) and consultative work as branches of the psychodynamic tree.

Amid all this, what is psychoanalysis? And who are the psychoanalysts? Psychoanalysis, which is synonymous with the theories of Sigmund Freud (1856–1939), Moravian physician and neurologist, relates to psychodynamic theory in roughly the way Darwinism relates to biology. It is not the whole story, and is not without controversy, but it is one of several fundamental tenets. You could classify psychotherapists into behaviour therapists (including cognitive behaviour therapists) and psychodynamic therapists although, as we have indicated elsewhere in this book, they use different models. The latter make use of psychoanalytic principles, and of them only a proportion will be psychoanalytically trained. Of the

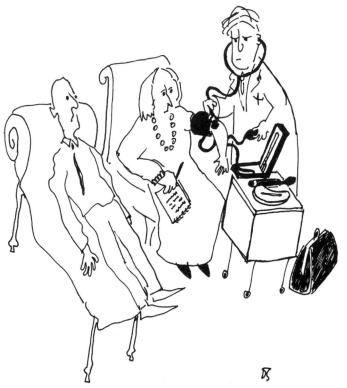

'psychoanalysis may be daily for several years'

psychoanalytically trained psychotherapists, only a proportion practise classical psychoanalysis, i.e. with the patient talking from a recumbent posistion on a couch, with the psychoanalyst spending most of the time listening.

Much psychoanalytic psychotherapy is conducted for training purposes (i.e. training other psychodynamic psychotherapists) but tends to be known nonetheless as 'being in therapy' by these trainees, which is a confusing notion. We consider training one thing, therapy another. Dynamic psychotherapy can be on a weekly basis for a few weeks or months; psychoanalysis may be daily for several years. Between these extremes are many variations.

Another feature of psychodynamic therapy for the purposes of this general introduction is the concept of supervision. The average house physician or house surgeon arrives on the first day of the first job with his bleep going as he struggles into a starched white coat, and supposedly knows everything. In a week or so there will be a ward round where the houseman is politely interrogated by the consultant about the surviving patients. The professional undertaking *kosher* psychodynamic psychotherapy, however, is expected until very experienced indeed, and perhaps into early middle age, to take his or her work to a psychodynamic psychotherapist for supervision, at which, session by session, every utterance of patient and therapist, every non-verbal action (e.g. being late, a yawn, a period of silence) is gone into for the light it may throw on the patient, the problem, the progress of the work and *the therapist*.

IS IT TRUE? DOES IT WORK?

There is a great deal of truth in psychodynamic notions, but it is not the whole truth. It is also true that again and again it defies attempts to 'prove' it is effective, because 'it' varies so much, and it is difficult to define objective criteria for progress. On the one hand clinicians who pay attention to what their patients say and do and to their own personal reactions will find an intriguing face validity in the psychodynamic way of looking at things. On another hand, spending time attending to the meanings and feelings behind the superficial words of people in difficulties is, in the words of a pragmatic and distinguished practitioner, 'a very civilized, humane service offered to another human being' (Wilson 1986). Yet, on the third hand, psychodynamic psychotherapy is time-consuming and therefore expensive, and too easy, in a liberal, well-meaning sort of way, to suggest for everybody, even those who would be better off with, say, medication or behaviour therapy. Nonetheless it is ridiculous simply to dismiss it as rubbish. (Interestingly, to do so illustrates the angry use of a metaphor for encapsulating the notion of dirt, dust, junk and other unwanted stuff best thrown away, which is precisely the sort of combination of real feelings plus usable abstractions with which psychodynamicists work.)

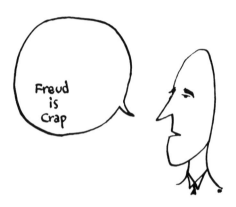

BASICS

Here are a few basic assumptions, or fundamental principles, which illustrate how a psychodynamic psychotherapist thinks.

Principle 1

His (or her) interest and clinical business is how the patient's patterns of thinking, feeling and behaving have got him into difficulties.

Principle 2

He (or she) cannot tell you immediately what these patterns of experience are, because they are a complex mixture of things valued, things disliked, things only partially grasped, and things so elusive that they cannot be put into words at all. And when they *are* put into words, the words seem inadequate not only intellectually but in terms of the feelings behind them. Moreover, both thoughts and feelings may be contradictory: the patient may like and dislike, or love and fear, certain people, things or situations, and would need the skills of an accomplished poet or novelist to convey them with any felicity (see Principle 10).

Principle 3

It takes time and mental exploration to begin to convey these things. It also takes a trusting relationship in which the patient can feel comfortable enough to become aware of and admit to *himself*, let alone anyone else, a range of thoughts, doubts and mixed feelings. These may include feeling sexual attraction or burning resentment (or both) towards his or her relations, friends, *et al.*, doubts about personal abilities, ambitions of cosmic proportions, or other such unworthy or manic ideas. All this takes time, and because it can be tricky and uncomfortable, and in a sense undisciplined (i.e. chaotic, unsystematic, uncensored) it works best within a definitely agreed framework. Thus whatever does or does not go on within a session, it is for a fixed period at a definite and regular time and place. The rules of time and place provide the safe structure within which decidedly unsafe matters can be explored. Any other sort of clinician may give popular patients frequent, long appointments and unpopular ones infrequent, short ones. The psychotherapist has technical reasons for keeping it the same come what may. (Can you believe that a sophisticated person might fear his therapist did not like him if, after he was mildly critical of her, she postponed the next appointment? But such things can happen, and are allowed for in the psychotherapist's technology.)

Principle 4

The latter points to a most important and fundamental assumption: that in general the ideas and feelings that mess people up are a little like free radicals in chemistry, that is they tend to attach themselves to other people, or more precisely *colour the image of the other person* and therefore affect the relationship. Thus suppose your patient has reasons in his psyche to tend to be paranoid. This paranoia (used here as a portmanteau term for any number of complex and subtle feelings) may have emerged in a relationship with a parent, become part of his repertoire in growing up, influenced his relationship with his wife, got in the way in relationships at work, and now (after the honeymoon period of therapy is over, during which you were the nice, kind therapist) *attaches itself to you*. This is the essence of *transference*, and goes well beyond the popular conception of 'falling in love with the analyst'. The wish to murder the therapist is more likely, and more useful. It is this immediate resurrection of old relationships with which the therapist works. Which are the 'real' feelings? Characteristically there can be real but opposing feelings, ie. *ambivalence*.

Principle 5

How are you to know that such feelings are there? The patient may well not tell you, particularly in the early stages, sometimes later, or sometimes never. The experienced therapist is alert to his or her own feelings towards the patient. The whole point of the dynamic psychotherapist having a training which gives psychodynamic insight is that such feelings of his own will be examined as objectively as possible; the philosopher and psychiatrist Henri Ey gave this important notion (the objective observation of subjective feelings) philosophical and clinical respectability (Evans 1972). It is important to appreciate that intellectual insight is not enough; the powerful, mixed and varying feelings that the patient in due course beams towards anyone who listens for long enough can be unnerving, boring or infuriating. This important phenomenon is known as *projection*, and how the process makes you feel is called the *countertransference*. If you cannot manage such feelings, tickled up in you by the patient, you may wish to pursue him out of the consulting room and down the stairs, or indeed precede him. Or, more likely, you may pick up and react to more subtle personal feelings, for example that the patient may feel so hopeless that he makes you feel that he is not only beyond help, and moreover not worth helping, but that you are not much good either.

All this may be true. But, at least in theory, a training which helps you use psychodynamic models aims to help you respond on the level, rather than trying too hard or giving up too soon. Another example, perhaps closer to home medically speaking, relates to dependency among patients. Built into the traditional socio-cultural position of the doctor is the powerful notion of needing a strong figure with magical powers when faced with illness, pain and death or the fear of death. The need to help can influence one person's career choice as a doctor just as it can another's career choice as patient. Feelings of dependency and the counter-feeling of protectiveness may emerge in a clinical relationship in an unhelpful way, so that a patient's unconscious need to be looked after is matched by the doctor's unconscious need to look after others. The patient becomes chronic and the clinic overloaded.

Principle 6

The *amorality* of psychodynamic thinking has often caused misunderstanding. The above account of the patient needing care and the doctor wishing to give it is not supposed to illustrate something good or bad, but just the way human beings operate. The dependent patient is no more 'bad' than the solicitous physician is 'good'. Rather, in an ideal world, doctor and patient would have enough grasp of the emotional side of their mutual relationship to keep the relationship at an appropriate and helpful level; 'good enough', to adapt the psychoanalyst D.W. Winnicott's term for the parent who gets the balance about right between, among other things, overprotectiveness and underprotectiveness (Winnicott 1974, 1991).

Principle 7

By the same token, you will understand a great deal about the psychodynamic model if you appreciate that in these vignettes we are not suggesting that there are 'out there' armies of dependent patients and overprotective clinicians, quite unlike sensible people like ourselves, but that tendencies toward such feelings are universal. The psychodynamic model suggests that such tendencies to incline in one direction (e.g. dependence, paranoia, sadness) or another (e.g. independence, trust, euphoria) are components of the psychology of all of us, and the points of balance shift and vary with different people in different circumstances and relationships at different times. Hence we can understand, if not agree with, the proclamation by Peter Simple's Dr Kiosk that 'we are all guilty'. It is when a particular frame of mind tends to predominate and endure regardless of the real circumstances that, if it is distressing or handicapping, it can become identified as a neurosis (which is short for psychoneurosis) and it *may* then be amenable to one of the dynamic psychotherapies.

We could sum up the story so far by saying that the essence of the psychodynamic model is that things are not necessarily what they seem. The 'nice' person may 'invest' in niceness (initially) because they are busy managing paranoid feelings, or the 'happy' person may be coping well with sadness. These balancing acts may be (a) integral to normal human functioning or (b) decompensate into something neurotic and disturbing.

The notion of the *unconscious* is fundamental to the concept of unperceived feelings, and to the psychodynamic models. The unconscious is hard to discuss without reaching for misleading

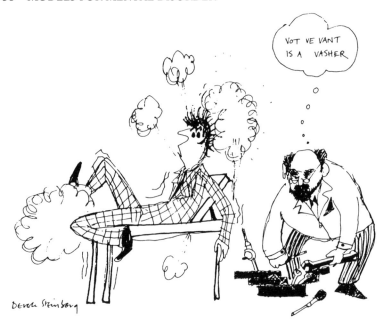

'. . . leaking out like molten lava or a burst pipe . . .'

analogies. In Freud's time, when 19th century physics and engineering were at their peaks, the models for that which was beyond verbal description tended to be geological or hydraulic: pressures from within, held down by powerful forces, diverted by valves, leaking out like molten lava or a burst pipe, were the metaphors of the day. In an earlier time demons, angels and similar beings up there or down below were invoked for explaining the inexplicable. More recently models for the mind have tended towards electronic circuits. At present we are moving into the quantum physics and chaos theory mode, and we may well wonder about the conceptual models of the future. An example of a model that misleads is the hydrodynamic, 'pressure cooker' model of stress, which may make people interpret uncomfortable feelings as internal forces that must be 'let out' one way or another. The relationship between such concepts and effective treatments is unclear.

A simpler concept for the 'unconscious', and one consistent with much psychodynamic thinking and therapy, connects conscious and observable verbal and non-verbal signals (words plus the minutiae of social behaviour) with internal feelings and images. Presented with any simple or complex stimulus (e.g. a phrase, an image or the first perception of another person) we can pursue a train of thought which can lead in unexpected directions. It may make unexpected connections, 'lighting up' pleasant or unwelcome images and associated feelings, some relevant, some irrelevant, or make the day-dreamer become alert with a start as something urgent and forgotten is recalled; perhaps the promise to make a phone call. It is likely that the sort of verbal connections that happen when one *free associates* in this way (the term and technique are those of the Swiss psychiatrist and psychoanalyst C.G. Jung) have some neurophysiological and neurochemical representation in the brain tracts and synaptic connections. It is also likely that such connections range from the entirely random, through those more or less habitual, to some predisposed by anatomy and evolution, and some triggered by matters currently important in our mental lives. It is also probable that countless such connections are being made, interconnected and broken all the time as part of the brain's life and alertness, precipitated by stimuli from within and without which range from the most trivial (the feel of your bottom on the chair, now) to something more imperative (e.g. a knock at the door, or an idea for a novel). The buzzing brain, and its part in modulating the sympathetic, parasympathetic and endocrine systems, is likely to contain much that is quite inaccessible except in certain circumstances (e.g. relaxation, dreaming, psychoanalysis) and some that is easily available if we 'turn our minds' to it. This may be a more valid model than the idea of inner pressures or a murky dark sea in which strange denizens ('complexes') are imagined to swim or lurk.

Whatever model is preferred, however, the unifying idea is of substantial mental activity continuing outside our awareness, yet at the same time being able to influence our awareness. Opponents of the concept of the unconscious mind have suggested that the very notion is illogical—that something unconscious cannot be part of the mind. They may have a point in that unconscious *thought* is perhaps an oxymoronic concept, but there is nothing inherently unsound in the notion of our thoughts and feelings being influenced by, or even driven by, psychophysiological processes from within.

Principle 8

Given this constant inner activity, we return again to the concept of the process being a dynamic one. Water may be at a constant level because of a balance between what flows in, what flows out and evaporation. (To adapt an ancient saying, you may have fond recollections of a stretch of water, indeed value its constancy, yet you can never step into the same stream twice.) Mental life has a constancy and rhythm, but the inner images, feelings and attitudes that constitute our moods and personalities are constantly being fed by perceptions from outside (traumatic, 'ordinary' and therapeutic) and no doubt by underground streams and fluctuating water tables too. But we digress into metaphors again.

Be all this as it may, such processes are not entirely random. The developing, maturing brain modulates itself, so that up to a point it 'hears what it wants to hear', and copes by keeping a balance between that which will fit in with existing beliefs and feelings and that which will upset the apple cart. Such defensive, adaptive processes, known as the *mechanisms of defence* were part of classical Freudian theory, but developed further by Freud's daughter Anna (Freud 1936).

One example is *rationalization*. Earlier, we painted the picture of clinician and patient becoming thoroughly fed up (note the metaphor) with each other, indeed sick of each other. Nevertheless, it is possible not only to imagine the mutual courtesies with which the final appointment and the re-referral to someone else is arranged, but also the inner feelings on both sides that these practical steps are wholly positive, sensible and civilized; what a good doctor, patient, indeed clinic, and how nice we all are.

Another is *denial*, the insistence that something isn't so when it very obviously is ('I am *not* angry!!') and another is *repression*, when something is pushed firmly out of our awareness because it threatens psychological homeostasis. *Projection* has already been described. *Reaction formation* is a very nice example, when a forbidden drive that is taboo (for the individual, the community or usually both) is converted within into acceptable currency; thus the extreme solicitousness, albeit on a short fuse, of the irritable restauranteur— or doctor.

Principle 9

These and other vastly complex processes proceed not only in *inner* homeostatic activity which tends to protect from unmanageable pain or distress, but in an *outer* social process too. (Thus the therapist and patient parting amicably in the above example is all right. The alternatives were (a) the therapist understanding and deciding to *work through** the countertransference, or (b) not understanding

* another technical term.

what was going on sufficiently to handle the situation properly and getting into a destructive fight with the patient.)

Thus to this picture of hidden depths within the individual we should add the hidden depths within the *interaction*, as one set of hidden depths communicates with the other.

('I really must go' says the long-staying guest, leaning back in the armchair; 'What a shame, must you really?' asks the hostess, leaping to her feet. Consider the layers of feeling within each, *and* in the social interaction.)

At a more aesthetic level, it is intriguing to consider what artists and composers may have put into their work even centuries ago, and which now conveys something to the observer or listener, yet which neither creator nor appreciator could put into words.

Principle 10

We referred earlier to the need for creative skills if the ambiguous, contradictory and only half-perceived in our minds was to be grasped and communicated. Human beings are extraordinarily inventive, and the unique capacity for language is partly to do with the capacity to transform images and feelings into sounds and symbols which convey something of those images and feelings to others. We see this capacity for symbolism and non-verbal expression in some symptoms (page 48).

In the above 10 examples of fundamental principles of psychodynamic thinking we have used analogies from ordinary life as well as from the clinic. This represents the idea of psychodynamic psychology having much to say about the whole of mental life, normal, abnormal and borderline. However, the essence of psychodynamic psychotherapy is to recognize those processes, within the individual and reflected in the relationship, which are causing distress and handicap, and to try to change them. How to do so is beyond the scope and purpose of this book; but we will not be daunted, and will try to outline in three sentences the essence of psychodynamic psychotherapy. First, the patient accepts at a rational, intellectual, cognitive level that he or she has a problem amenable to therapy based on conversation. This gradually changes to an emotionally-laden relationship with the therapist within which feelings and attitudes *about the self and the therapist* can be identified, explored, and sorted into those worth keeping and those best let go. The patient is thereby enabled to become a different person within the therapeutic relationship, and the whole of the argument about whether or not psychodynamic psychotherapy 'works' rests upon whether or not he or she continues to be a different person outside it.

VARIATIONS ON THE THEME

Psychodynamic psychology is represented by an enormously rich literature and body of ideas which extends into many quite different types of clinical theory and practice, and outwards into the sciences, religion and the arts. For our limited purposes, to convey something of the variety, breadth and depth of the field, we will select fragments of different schools of thought.

Freud

From Sigmund Freud, we may draw attention to the crucial pleasure and pain principles, by which the organism is drawn towards that which gratifies and away from that which is less pleasurable and more painful. This reminds us of the amoeba; and of Le Gros Clark's maxim that the first sign of life is irritability (Clark, 1947). It is also a reminder that first and foremost Freud was a biological thinker, who believed that the neurophysiology of the future would support his theories (Sulloway 1979).

Freudian theory is probably best known for its division of mental life into the *ego*, the *superego* and the *id*. We start with the *id*, in translation the 'it', a bundle of primitive instincts and impulses without direction or guidance beyond moving towards gratification on the pleasure–pain continuum. From this movement 'it' begins to learn something about external reality, and part of the *id* becomes differentiated into the self, and ultimately the self-conscious self, or ego. An important part of this reality is the social reality developed by other people, the expectations, rules and taboos in the family, the community and the culture in which the ego develops, and with which the ego has to come to terms. This adoption of 'the rules' by the developing individual makes up its super-ego, which very roughly is like his or her conscience. It largely picks up the rules, partly unconsciously, partly with mixed feelings (ambivalence again) from *identification* with parents or parent-figures by a process known as *introjection* ('taking on board', in the modern managerial parlance). As might well be imagined, there follows a great deal of struggling between the needs of the *id*, the dictates of the super-ego and the wishes of the ego, which by their psychodynamic interaction achieve a degree of homeostasis. If they do not, the individual or the community suffers. One fundamental task for the infant male to tackle, according to Freud, is how to cope with the discovery that another male, and indeed a big, strong one, has an interest in his own first love, his mother. This could be dangerous, and represents the discovery of a love and sex that invited punishment, i.e. incest. This is the basic model for the distinguished *Oedipal complex*, the resolution of which (i.e. the coming to terms with) was regarded by Freud as a necessary challenge for boys. He was less clear about girls.

Freud is also known for his attention to dreams, the 'royal road to the unconscious'. His book *The Interpretation of Dreams* is worth reading as a gripping work of literature, whatever else it is. In brief the psychoanalytic thesis is that dreams are charged with meaning. Physiological studies of sleep and dreaming confirm that dreaming, including the contents of dreams, has some function, but not particularly that which lends itself convincingly to Freudian interpretation. A reasonable view is that as far as the brain is concerned, life goes on day and night rather as sketched on page 39, with events that include the random, the emotionally significant, *and* those which the individual can make useful stories from (as from cloud patterns) when awake, e.g. with his psychoanalyst.

A good, short account of Freudian ideas and those which derive from them is to be found in Brown (1961). An important reminder that Freud was trying to convey complex, subtle meanings that were not always adequately translated will be found in Bettelheim (1985). Two valuable and much larger works are by Wyss (1966) and Ellenberger (1970).

Attachment theory is a more recent development which makes connections between psychoanalytic thinking, human relationships and our knowledge of animal behaviour (especially primates) and provides interesting models for symptom-formation. It is described on page 46. It is an example of the relatively new science of ethology, which is concerned with the evolution, purpose and meaning of behaviour.

Jung

A whole school of psychodynamic psychology (known officially as analytical psychology) was developed by the Swiss psychiatrist C.G. Jung (1875–1961). If Freudian theory is in a sense psychobiological in its roots, Jungian theory is more based in cultural anthropology and mythology, although again with roots in social biology. Perhaps its most significant departure, or discovery, is the concept of the *collective unconscious*, and unconscious 'images' or potential images within it known as the *archetypes* of the collective unconscious. These intriguing ideas have been widely misunderstood to refer to all sorts of alarming and provocative notions such as racial memories (inherited by some sort of discredited Lamarckian process) and mass telepathy, and to be fair to Jung's critics it may be said that some of his writing is contradictory and unclear on these and other themes. However, it is well established by anthropologists and others that there are as many similarities as differences in the patterns of human behaviour and artistic and religious productions, even when there is no evidence of historical contact between various human groups. It is not far-fetched to suppose that the human imagination may have evolved within a developing human culture just as everything else about us has evolved, and that some inner fantasies and fancies e.g. of gods, demons and big bad monsters may be shared in common. A rewarding account of Jung from the biological perspective, without detracting from others, will be found in Stevens (1982).

If Freudian psychotherapy *tends* towards the interpretation of unconscious material to do with sex, death and self-assertion, very much around the Oedipal theme and in the patient's own life, and with the patient doing most of the talking to a characteristically non-committal analyst, then Jungian therapy tends towards the conversational, the universal rather than the reductionist, and to the individual's roots in his or her background and culture rather than in animal origins. Jungian therapists are also more inclined to use art techniques in therapy, e.g. painting and drawing. But, we emphasize, these are stereotypes, and there are as many types of practice as there are practitioners.

Adler

Alfred Adler (1870–1937), once the third great figure in the analytical trinity, has been relatively neglected in recent years. He founded individual psychology and we owe to him the concept of the *inferiority complex* and how disabilities can be compensated for in both neurotic and productive ways. His theories, and the practice deriving from them, are more reality-orientated and to do with setting goals, self-management and so on. He may return.

Klein

The ideas of Melanie Klein (1882–1960) can be baffling and to some have been infuriating, but one concept is particularly interesting and valuable and can show the way into a wider appreciation of her work. This is an elaboration of the notion of the ego's struggle (see above) in a period when the infant cannot distinguish between itself and the reality 'outside'. Feeling good (when gratified for example by food and warmth) and feeling bad (when these things are absent) are attributed (projected) as outside phenomena, 'good objects' and 'bad objects'. The former are the objects of the infant's intense love, to be totally taken in, and the latter are the objects of hatred, to be destroyed or at least controlled. The primitive feelings developing at this stage 'in a world peopled by gods and devils' (Brown 1961) was termed the *paranoid position*, and a very instructive position it is if you allow that psychodynamic ideas about infants might throw light on political as well as clinical positions.

But there is more to this account. In due course the child makes a painful and formative discovery: that the object of its love, and of its hatred, are one and the same—the sometimes-gratifying and sometimes-nongratifying mother. The child is still immature enough to believe in magic, that his love can preserve his mother and his hate can destroy her, and he is in a confused and ambivalent position. From this he can *regress* to the comforts of the paranoid position (where everything is good or bad, black or white), or try to make sense of his new discovery, which is a depressing experience (nothing's quite that simple; wait; be patient, put up with it; persevere) known as the *depressive position*. In Kleinian theory, and in therapy informed by its principles, the experience and acceptance of depression represents progress and a maturational step forwards, as indeed it can be in life outside therapy.

Klein described all this in terms of the mental life of the child in the first two or three months. It is easy for Klein's critics and proponents to become caught up on the argument (often, a blazing row) about whether anyone could know anything so specific about so young an infant, still less whether it can be of use, as Klein believed, in psychotherapy for children. And yet a look at human affairs in the newspapers or closer to home suggests that this model of infantile behaviour and its consequences has a heuristic value and a degree of clinical validity.

SYMPTOM FORMATION

Psychodynamic theory is stronger on the general causes of human distress and the results of problems or breakdown in relationships than on the explanation of specific symptoms. Thus in Kleinian terms the psychodynamic model provides a possible explanation for

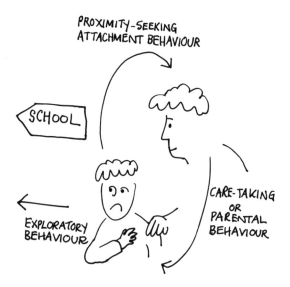

Fig 3.1

anger and depression when reality intrudes on an over-dependent relationship. The Freudian model can explain some patterns of anxiety and guilt when someone with problems in self-esteem and self-confidence feels they have over-asserted themselves in general, or in a particular relationship, and expect and fear retribution. In such psychodynamic explanations of symptoms there is the assumption that intense feelings belonging to childhood can be reactivated when someone is under pressure and in emotional and perhaps behavioural terms too he or she *regresses*.

An interesting model for regression derives from *attachment theory*, really a set of models and theories developed by John Bowlby (Bowlby 1969, 1973, 1980) which link psychodynamic concepts, parent–child behaviour and animal (especially primate) behaviour. Figure 3.1 gives a simplified model of a dynamic interaction between a dependent child and a care-taking adult, with the child's *proximity-seeking attachment behaviour* (e.g. crying, 'attention seeking', etc.) balanced by 'good enough' parenting or *caretaking behaviour* so that the child is neither neglected nor overprotected, and can therefore undertake the sort of *exploratory* behaviour that is expected in children and biologically necessary in human development. If the child's attachment behaviour does not trigger sufficient care-taking behaviour (because of a problem on either or both sides

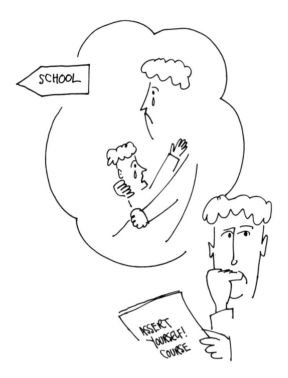

Fig 3.2

of the relationship) it tries, so the model goes, the behaviour that worked 'before', i.e. when the child was younger. Thus a plea, then nagging, then crying, all falling on deaf ears so to speak, might lead the child to regress to previous ways of eliciting a reaction, such as screaming, misbehaviour or complaining of stomach ache or feeling sick.

The same model provides a descriptive explanation of the means by which experiences become incorporated in the developing personality (*introjection* again). Figure 3.2 conveys the event becoming incorporated as an experience (or more likely set of experiences, and therefore assumptions about parenting), so that the child grows up with a tendency to expect the worst, feel anxious, not to trust, have a low self-esteem or to have somatic symptoms when anxious. Hence also behaviour within the family system, and perhaps amenable to family therapy, becomes part of the individual's own repertoire as an individual disorder needing individual treatment.

There is little evidence of a single 'traumatic experience' being behind the development of neuroses and maladaptive personality traits. Children are quite resilient. Rather it is the accumulation of such negative experiences in a persisting pattern of youthful problems and parental mishandling that establishes feelings and behaviours we later describe as psychiatric conditions. Attachment theory provides some illuminating models for this.

Parkes (1969) provides similar socio-psychodynamic models. These demonstrate the similarities between the depressive symptoms of grief, the similar symptoms following amputation and other losses, and the actual behaviour of young humans and primates when separated from parents, with 'grieving' behaviour in the latter. Here biological observations tend to confirm the psychoanalytic metaphor of the 'search for a lost object'.

Hysteria (originally attributed to the uterus wandering about the body) remains a puzzle. It may be defined as the resort to *symbolic* problems when, for some reason, the direct expression of anxiety or distress is blocked. This may be due to immaturity, cultural convention, to another aspect of neurotic personality structure (e.g. denial at all costs) or due to the situation being extraordinarily difficult. In recent years for example many psychiatrists have begun to see hysterical behaviour such as simulated physical disability (e.g. paralysis, inability to swallow) in young people with a history of sexual abuse. Sometimes this takes the form of such chaotic thinking and behaviour that the condition is described as a reactive psychosis.

Anorexia nervosa is intriguing in this respect. Whatever its likely multiple bio-psychosocial origins, a psychodynamic formulation sometimes provides compelling reasons why the girl (incidentally, 10% of patients are male) does not want to grow up, and appears to have the uncanny knack of holding back her weight at just the point where menstruation ceases.

Anxiety or depression may be associated with phobic symptoms which include a wish to escape from the scene or a fear of falling; again, the problem may be low self-esteem, shame or fear of failure, expressed as a fear of being seen to fall in public. The language is full of such metaphors—the fallen woman, 'collapse of stout party' and so on. This is hardly surprising; the language of illness and the language of literature from soap operas to operas comes from the same source. (As of course does the language of psychoanalysis.)

This universality of symbolic expression obscures as much as it illuminates. The patient with a sense that something has gone wrong within him and of developing psychic incapacity may express his feelings in classical psychoanalytic terms. He may have a classical psychoanalytic problem, or a disorder of the chemistry which maintains normal moods, or a neurodegenerative disorder. The woman who feels weak and dizzy and dreams of being caught undressed in the street may have a neurosis, a personality problem or anaemia. None of this invalidates the psychodynamic model for some patients, or some aspects of some patients.

PRACTICAL APPLICATIONS

The content and implications of psychodynamic theory tend to be protean, as well they might, considering that it comprises a highly variegated but universal model for human mental life, and involves biology, social science, anthropology, religion and the arts in its psychology.

Not surprisingly, you could derive quite different areas of work and forms of practice from different aspects of a patchwork which has had so many contributions over the past hundred years.

Individual psychoanalysis still stands, or lies, with the *analysands* going five times a week for a couple of years for their 'first' analysis, although we understand a second analysis can be as *de rigueur* as a farmhouse in France. The indications for psychoanalysis as treatment are not for discussion here, but, as mentioned earlier, it is understandable that a training analysis is appropriate for psychotherapists who intend to practise psychoanalysis or psychoanalytic psychotherapy, as a necessary aid to clear thinking and appropriate responses when the projections begin to fly.

This is a reminder (from the ever-helpful unconscious) that we forgot all about *Freudian slips*. There was a beautiful example during the 1992 Conservative Party Conference when a senior UK politican was being interviewed about what Margaret Thatcher was like to work with. He referred to blazing rows 'when she would hit the fan'*. Like dreams, Freudian slips may be guided by significant feelings, or be entirely random, or due to other influences (e.g. the proximity of certain keys on the typewriter keybored) or by a combination of these things.

Pychodynamic psychotherapy is systematic psychotherapy guided by psychodynamic principles, in which the practitioner may be thoroughly trained or hardly trained at all, and may be practically indistinguishable from psychoanalysis at one end of the spectrum, to hardly recognizable at all as psychotherapy at the other. The field

---

* readers who do not understand the joke are invited to apply to the authors for an explanation.

is that variable; but within it there is much highly skilled, dedicated work of the highest integrity.

Precisely the same is true of a vast range of *creative* or *'humanistic'*, and *'progressive'* psychotherapies, and those with a special focus such as marital relationships and sex. Here psychotherapy and counselling blur into each other, although one might define the former as being concerned with fundamental change in feelings and the latter more to do with advice, practical management and self-management.

Drama therapy and *art therapy* are forms of therapy where activity, such as acting roles or expressing feelings in paint and other art work, take precedence over words in establishing the therapeutic relationship and representing feelings. For children, *play therapy* is a technique with similarities. It may be supposed that they are particularly useful where the patient is less articulate; on the contrary, a patient with highly developed verbal skills may deal with feelings in too intellectual a way, and the techniques of art and drama can then usefully bypass overactive 'higher centres'. Jennings (1983) provides an excellent overview of the creative therapies in very practical terms, and Thomson (1989) an outstanding short guide to the principles of art therapy.

Family therapy, which itself contains many schools of thought and practice, is similarly concerned with actions more than words. The family therapies have more or less in common the principle that what is recalled in the 'one-to-one' or dyadic therapeutic session, is actually played out before the eyes of all concerned in family therapy. For example, if a boy forms a teasing alliance with his mother and excludes the father, who gets ever angrier, the family therapist might intervene with comments or actions. The therapist might invite the mother to move her position to where she can see her husband's reaction, and ask the father if he is happy with his son leaning his head on his mother's shoulder, and does he want to ask him to move? Family therapy may follow group analytic lines (i.e. psychoanalytic theory as applied to groups) or systemic theory.

The latter is an interesting model based on social systems theory rather than psychoanalytic theory; it represents a social rather than psychological dynamic, in that the system (e.g. a family group) reaches a particular state of homeostasis in which (for example) various roles become fixed, e.g. the misbehaving adolescent, the 'good' but depressed big sister, the workaholic husband and the alcoholic wife. The presenting symptom, or in family therapy parlance the identified patient, may be the naughty boy, but he may in some respects be the 'healthiest' family member, challenging the family's stability (unconsciously) to draw attention to a range of (denied) problems. The small boat with several people in it is quite a good model to understand family therapy; if one person changes position everyone else has to move, some more than others, to achieve stability again. In the process the presenting problems can diminish and others be identified. Family therapy has an enormous number of good introductory books, all different. One, by Robin Skynner and John Cleese (1984), nicely straddles individual and family dynamics.

From family therapy we are another step away from traditional psychodynamic theory and closer to *group and social theory*, with their counterparts not only in small group therapies (with some overlap with family therapy), but in the understanding of large

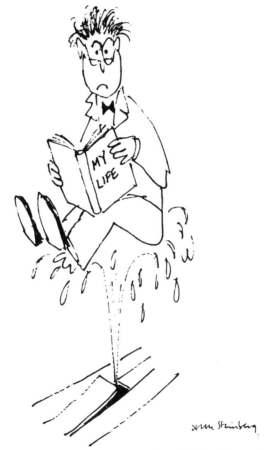

'. . . it is a long way from the simplistic hydraulic model'

groups too, including very large groups and groupings in organizations such as hospitals and other institutions (Kreeger 1975, Skynner 1989).

Here, on the outer edge of the psychodynamic universe, we enter another world, one pioneered by the Tavistock Institute in London, where the dynamics of the interaction not only between people and groups but between departments, agencies and professions has been explored (e.g. Caplan 1970, Steinberg 1989, Trist & Murray 1990). At this point we have gone full circle and are looking at models for social systems which foster, or fail to foster, individual development.

CONCLUSION

What is intriguing about psychodynamic theory is not that it is a rich mixture of the implausible and the commonsensical, the banal and the brilliant, but that many sensible people disagree over which is which. Taken overall, the special gift to the clinician of the psychodynamic model is not to help make oversimplified and ultimately wrong assumptions about psychosomatic disorders and other aspects of feelings and behaviour, but to appreciate the rich complexity of people's lives, our development and, ultimately, our evolution. It is against this biological and biographical background that the pain in the neck, or indeed in the backside, can be more fully understood; it is a long way from the simplistic hydraulic model.

REFERENCES

Bettelheim, B. (1985) *Freud and Man's Soul*. Fontana, London.

Bowlby, J. (1969) *Attachment and Loss. Volume 1: Attachment*, Hogarth Press, London.

Bowlby, J. (1973) *Attachment and Loss. Volume 2: Separation: Anxiety and Anger*. Hogarth Press, London.

Bowlby, J. (1980) *Attachment and Loss. Volume 3: Loss*. Hogarth Press, London.

Brown, J.A.C. (1961) *Feud and the Post-Freudians*. Penguin Books, Harmondsworth.

Caplan, G. (1970) *The Theory and Practice of Mental Health Consultation*. Tavistock, London.

Clark, Le Gros (1947) *The Tissues of the Body*. Cambridge University Press, Cambridge.

Ellenberger, H.F. (1970) *The Discovery of the Unconscious*. Allen Lane the Penguin Press, London.

Evans, P. (1972) Henri Ey's concepts of the organisation of consciousness and its disorganisation: an extension of Jacksonian theory. *Brain*, **95**, 2, 413–440.

Freud, A. (1936) *The Ego and the Mechanisms of Defence*. Hogarth Press, London.

Freud, S. (1954) *The Interpretation of Dreams*. Trans. J. Strachey, George Allen and Unwin, London.

Jennings, S. (1983) *Creative Therapy*. Kemble Press, Banbury.

Kreeger, L. (1975) *The Large Group*. Constable, London.

Parkes, C.M. (1969) Separation anxiety: an aspect of the search for a lost object. In *Studies of Anxiety* (ed) M.H. Lader. Royal Medico-Psychological Association, London.

Skynner, R. (1989) *Institutes and How to Survive Them*. (ed) J. Schlapobersky. Methuen, London.

Skynner, R. and Cleese, J. (1984) *Families and How to Survive Them*. Methuen, London.

Steinberg, D. (1989) *Interprofessional Consultation. Innovation and Imagination in Working Relationships*. Blackwell Scientific Publications, Oxford.

Stevens, A. (1982) *Archetype: a Natural History of the Self*. Routledge and Kegan Paul, London.

Sulloway, F.J. (1979) *Freud: Biologist of the Mind*. Andre Deutsch, London.

Thomson, M. (1989) *On Art and Therapy*. Virago, London.

Trist, E. and Murray, H. (1990) (eds) *The Social Engagement of Social Science. A Tavistock Anthology*. Volume 1: the Socio-psychological Perspective. Free Association Books, London.

Wilson, P. (1986) Individual psychotherapy in a residential setting. In *The Adolescent Unit* (ed) D. Steinberg, Wiley, Chichester.

Winnicott, D.W. (1974) *Playing and Reality*. Pelican, Harmondsworth.

Winnicott, D.W. (1991) *Human Nature*. Free Association Books, London.

Wyss, D. (1966) *Depth Psychology. A Critical History*. George Allen and Unwin, London.

CHAPTER 4

The Behavioural Model

'Freudian theory regards neurotic symptoms as "the visible upshot of unconscious causes". Learning theory does not postulate any such "unconscious" causes, but regards neurotic symptoms as simply learned habits; there is no neurosis underlying the symptom but merely the symptom itself. Get rid of the symptom and you have eliminated the neurosis.'

H.J. Eysenck 1965

The behavioural model of mental illness adopts a fundamentally different approach from the biological, psychodynamic and social models. This is seen most starkly in their respective views of mental symptoms. The psychotherapist regards his patients' symptoms as presenting features that obscure and mislead rather than edify or explain. He regards symptoms as not just the tip of an iceberg but as a decoy iceberg that is separated from its complete submerged partner. If the symptoms are treated directly they will only reappear in another form (symptom substitution) and so they should be regarded as clues to the underlying problem but having no real substance. The biological psychiatrist differs in finding symptoms useful as components of syndromes but does not in general regard them as primary phenomena. Similarly, the social psychiatrist looks on symptoms as culturally determined reactions to social forces that have no special significance in themselves.

The behavioural model looks no further than the symptoms, which, together with the behaviour that follows from them, *are* the disorder. The symptoms develop through a process of learning, or conditioning, and because they are unhelpful they are described as maladaptive learned responses. It is helpful, but not essential, for the therapist to find out how the maladaptive learning has developed because this may decide the best form of treatment. Learning goes on all the time but is usually appropriate and therefore adaptive. The distressing symptoms of mental disorder develop when the subject has missed the cues that help him to adapt. He is like a traveller who has lost his way after taking a wrong turning. The job of the therapist is to help him to retrace his steps or take a new route to the correct way again (counter-conditioning).

Learning theory is a psychological science that has an excellent pedigree. Two forms of conditioning are responsible for the formation of symptoms, *classical* and *operant* conditioning. Classical conditioning refers to learning which takes place when a neutral stimulus becomes associated with a previously unrelated sequence of a stimulus and response. The reader will note that stimulus and response are directly linked; one follows from the other in the behavioural model without any complicated processes intervening. The psychotherapist finds this omission of mental processes profoundly distasteful, but the behaviourist retorts that the facts support his model. Classical conditioning was first described by the Russian physiologist, Pavlov in a celebrated series of experiments with dogs, first carried out with salivation. Dogs (and other mammals) salivate when eating. Having a plentiful supply of saliva helps in chewing food and also aids digestion as saliva contains enzymes which break down some of the food. Salivation normally starts when the dog smells the food so that by the time the first mouthful is taken there is saliva already secreted. All this makes good physiological sense and was known many years before Pavlov's experiments. The stimulus of food is followed by the response of salivation.

Pavlov introduced measurement to this phenomenon by cannulating the salivary ducts of the dogs so that the exact quantity of saliva could be recorded. He was then able to see if other stimuli altered salivary flow. By itself, the sound of a bell had no effect on salivary flow. But if the bell was sounded at or about the same time food was presented to the dog, after several trials the sound of the bell alone was enough to produce a copious flow of saliva. In other words, the neutral stimulus of the bell ringing had become linked to the stimulus (food)—response (salivation) and thereby had become a conditional stimulus. Now on the surface this experiment does not appear to be a breakthrough. The results probably could be predicted correctly by many who had no pretensions to special knowledge in the biological sciences. Indeed, the animal lover, Bernard Shaw, speaking as usual through the mouths of his characters, says

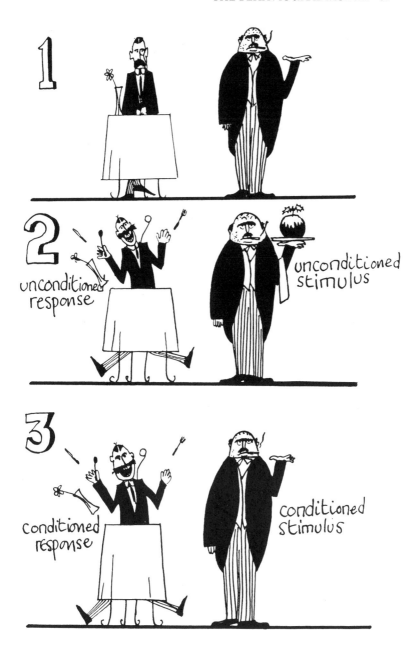

'The stimulus of food is followed by the response of salivation'

of this experiment*, 'Why didn't you ask me? I could have told you in 25 seconds without hurting those poor dogs'. Where Pavlov broke entirely new ground was in his detailed study of the factors which increase (positively reinforce) or reduce (negatively reinforce and, ultimately, extinguish) the conditioned response. The greater the frequency and the closer the bell and food were presented together in time, the stronger was the conditioning. Further experiments showed that when the dogs were put under stress their conditioned responses became disturbed. For example, a dog that had been conditioned to salivate in response to a circle but not to an ellipse displayed increasing signs of agitation when the ellipse was changed gradually until it was almost circular. Anxiety and agitation inhibit salivation and even when the dog was capable of making the correct choice salivary flow was not as great as formerly. Eventually Pavlov was able to produce a comprehensive physiological theory of abnormal behaviour based entirely on his experiments with classical conditioning (Pavlov 1927, 1941).

Operant conditioning differs from classical conditioning in that behaviour determines conditioning, not the stimulus. The psychologist, B.F. Skinner, the father of operant conditioning (Skinner 1972) and the Skinner box, which he invented, is one of the best methods of illustrating it in practice. A Skinner box consists of a closed box with one or more buttons, levers or switches which can be operated by an animal placed in the box. If a hungry pigeon is put in the box it will not at first have any stimulus-response patterns to reinforce so conditioning will not occur. However, in the course of exploring its new environment it is likely to peck at one of the buttons at the side of the box. If this is the correct button a small amount of food will be delivered into the box from a hopper outside. After gobbling this up the pigeon wants more. He does not know how the food arrived but before long he links the pecking of the button with the arrival of food. Once this is learnt the button will be pecked repeatedly until his appetite is satisfied. In this case positive reinforcement of the conditioned response (pecking the button) will be increased by the continual supply of food and extinguished by ceasing to provide food when the button is pecked. Unlike classical conditioning, which depends on the experimenter manipulating a neutral stimulus so that it becomes a conditioned one, operant conditioning is determined by the animal's own behaviour. If the pigeon shows no exploratory behaviour when it is put in the Skinner box it will not be conditioned.

---

* In *The Adventure of the Black Girl in Her Search for God.*

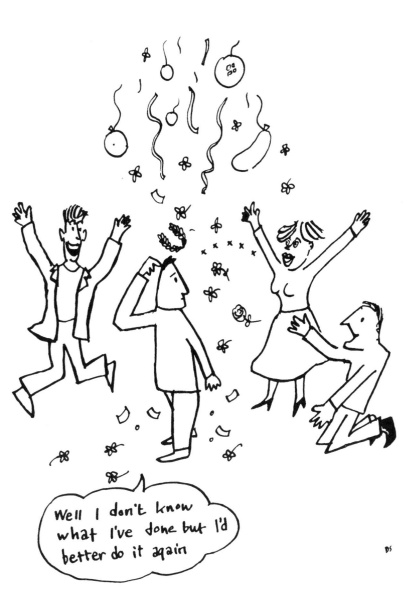

'. . . operant conditioning is determined by the animal's own behaviour'

These experiments of Skinner and Pavlov are so well known that you may wonder why we have described them in any detail. We have done so because they emphasize two important points. First, the behavioural model is based on scientific experiment, and involves measurement which can be replicated (unlike psychodynamic theory) and, secondly, that the learning theory underpinning it is easily understood and involves no leaps into fantastic notions such as those of the unconscious mind. By concentrating on behaviour all the hidden variables of depth psychologies become unimportant. We measure what we observe, manipulate by experimental and develop testable theories from the results.

It is at this point that the psychotherapists, some cognitive therapists and many social psychiatrists start to get upset. How can one infer from these simple experiments with animals anything about man's thinking and behaviour? What right have the behaviourists to imply that man, the 'paragon of animals', is 'controlled' by simple laws of stimulus and response? Is not man capable of exercising his free will and forging his own destiny rather than being an automaton at the mercy of the maelstrom of surrounding stimuli that he cannot control or ignore? These criticisms are aimed at reductionism, the philosophical view that complex problems can be understood through examination of their simplest elements.

The behaviourist regards these questions as rhetorical and gets on with his task of investigation and measurement. Early evidence that the same types of conditioning occurred in man came from an experiment by the American psychologist, Watson and Rayner (1920). Watson repeatedly sounded a loud noise at the same time as a young boy was presented with a tame white rat, a classical conditioning experiment along the same line as Pavlov's. The young boy was frightened by the loud noise and, not surprisingly, came to associated this with the presence of the rat. He therefore became frightened of the rat. Such fear is regarded as unreasonable (although perhaps understandable in the circumstances of the experiment) as rats are harmless, and such irrational fears are called phobias. The boy's phobia of white rats soon developed to a phobia of all furry animals, a phenomenon called generalization by the behaviourists. Normally when a response is not reinforced it is extinguished, but a phobia initiated in this way tends to persist. This is because a phobia is dealt with commonly by behaviour which prevents exposure to the phobic stimulus (avoidance) and this reinforces the fear. Each time you avoid any situation because you think it will make you anxious the fear you attach to this situation will increase. This is how the pattern of maladaptive responses becomes established. The boy is conditioned to fear rats under the circumstances of the experiment. He tends to avoid rats so the fear is reinforced. Each time he is exposed to furry animals he feels frightened and runs away (conditioned avoidance response) so he never gets a chance to realize that laboratory-bred rats are really harmless.

To restore a normal response the maladaptive one has to be replaced with an adaptive pattern of behaviour. This can be done by removing the fear response gradually, through imagining or being exposed to different, carefully graded levels of the phobic stimulus while relaxed (*systematic desensitization*); or dramatically, by preventing avoidance (*flooding* or '*implosion*'). Desensitization and flooding can also be combined in gradual exposure to the phobic stimulus. Better response is obtained if the patient carries out the treatment programme in real life rather than imagination (exposure *in vivo*). In many ways desensitization is the reverse of acquisition of the phobia. Images or actual representations of the phobic stimuli are presented in order from a furry toy, to a rabbit and finally to a live rat during deep relaxation. Once the lowest phase in the hierarchy is completed by the toy evoking no fear, the next stage is taken in the same way.

This technique treatment was first described by Wolpe (1958) who thought that 'reciprocal inhibition' was the important ingredient. Phobic fear was inhibited by the presence of relaxation elsewhere. Reciprocal inhibition is now seldom mentioned in relationship to desensitization. It derives from neurology, as in order for one set of muscles in the body to contract the opposing set of muscles has to relax and this is automatically achieved by the nervous system. However this is not the explanation of behaviour therapy and in any case it contains too much of the biological model to be acceptable. It is better to conclude that the maladaptive phobic behaviour is counter-conditioned by the desensitization. In flooding, the phobic person is put in the situation that makes him most anxious, and is then prevented from escaping from it. The principle of treatment is explained in advance; escape from the fear only reinforces the idea that the situation is dangerous. If escape is prevented the person's level of anxiety goes up at first but falls later as he realizes that the terrible consequences he fears do not in fact happen. In exposure therapy the subject is encouraged to tackle the fears gradually. Instead of being flung in at the deep end he tests the water gradually, moving steadily down towards the deeper levels, extinguishing his anxiety as he goes. Of course it is important for the therapist to reinforce the idea that the phobia is unjustified and make sure that there is nothing in the experimental situation that might support or replace the fears with new ones. An excellent example of how not to desensitize a phobia of rats is described in the last pages of George Orwell's celebrated novel, *1984*, in which the hero, Winston Smith, is 'cleansed' of all his heretical ideas by going to 'Room 101', a dreadful place where each person's special fears are exploited by techniques that have long been known by the name of brainwashing. Winston has a specific phobia of rats and this is reinforced by the inquisition of Room 101 before a solution is offered by clever counter-conditioning. He comes to understand that all his fears can be healed by forgetting his past notions and believing that the head of state, Big Brother, is the fount of truth and knowledge. When he says simply 'I love Big Brother' his counter-conditioning is complete.

The treatment of phobias was one of the first applications of behaviour techniques derived from the laboratory, but many disorders thought to be 'illnesses' are now recognized to be abnormal behaviour. The repeated checking of the obsessional, the stuttering of the stammerer, the craving of the alcoholic, the indecent exposure of the exhibitionist, the overdoses of attempted suicide, and the aggressive behaviour of the delinquent are now all accepted forms of abnormal behaviour suitable for modification. The behaviourist rejects the implications of the biological model and dislikes the word 'patient' being applied to the sufferer from abnormal behaviour because of its passive connotations. A person's behaviour is part of his responsibility, not something that can be handed over to a doctor to be removed. The behavioural model respects the integrity of the individual, and in successful management the client is closely involved with all stages of therapy. This is in the therapist's interests because once the treatment has been started it will be maintained by the client, who will himself learn about the principles of behaviour modification during the progress of his condition. By monitoring his own sessions in the consulting room, he develops greater confidence and self-esteem.

Let us look at a typical case suitable for assessment and treatment to use in the behavioural model. The format remains the same as with the other models, with the therapist's comments being in italics.

CASE HISTORY

The Presenting Problem

A young married woman of 23 gives a history of being nervous and frightened about going out of doors since she married her 36-year-old husband four months ago. Her symptoms first started after she returned from honeymoon. She and her husband moved into their new house in a town 40 miles away from her old home where she had lived with her family. She is afraid to go out of the house alone and also feels uneasy travelling with other people apart from her husband. *She has agoraphobic symptoms but these disappear when her husband is with her. He makes her feel secure and allays her anxiety.* She also sometimes feels frightened when left in the house on her own. Because of these feelings she has become progressively more dependent on her husband who is a self-employed builder and decorator. He has been very tolerant of her handicap an takes his wife to work with him to reduce her anxiety and accompanies her whenever she goes out shopping. She has tried going out alone on many occasions but each time she has acute attacks of panic which prevent her from completing the journey. She now refuses to travel by bus or shop in supermarkets alone. *She has developed a conditioned avoidance response. She expects to feel frightened whenever she goes out to shops and therefore avoids it. Each time she avoids going out she reinforces the idea that there is some danger in stepping outside the home alone and therefore the phobia is strengthened.* Her husband is prepared to accompany her whenever necessary and although he is willing to do this she feels guilty about having to ask him and is sure he is irritated by her need to do so. She no longer feels as close to her husband as she did before. Matters have not been helped by her reduced sexual interest and at times she has been unable to complete sexual intercourse because of frigidity. *This is a secondary phenomenon. Her phobias have made her more anxious and insecure.* She now feels tense most of the time and always panics when she thinks of going out of the house. *Continued reinforcement of the phobia has increased its severity.*

Family and Personal History

Her mother has always been anxious and has had fears of travelling by train for many years. *Her daughter would almost certainly be aware of this and imitate her mother to some extent (modelling) in regarding such fears as reasonable and appropriate.* She is the younger of two sisters. Her elder sister, four years older, has been married for eight years but is having difficulties in her relationship with her husband and there is talk of separation. Her father was a regular army non-commissioned officer and was moved frequently during her childhood. This interrupted the patient's schooling and at times she had short episodes of refusing to go to school following transfer to a different part of the country. *These were the first signs of her adult phobic symptoms.* One of these episodes lasted for two weeks during which she had severe headaches and had episodes of vomiting and the school attendance officer had to be called in. According to her school reports she always underachieved at school and appeared to be uncomfortable there. She had few friends, passed no examinations and left, aged 15.

Previous Personality

She has always been an anxious, shy person and has found it difficult to make friends. The friends she has made have been very close and she has tended to rely on them a great deal. She prefers an ordered life and her hobbies include knitting and crocheting, crossword puzzles and watching television. She smokes 15 cigarettes a day. *This type of personality is prone to maladaptive conditioning. Once patterns of behaviour are established they are difficult to break.*

Mental State

At interview she presented as a carefully made-up young woman who was fairly anxious during interview and frequently smoothed back her hair and flicked imaginary pieces of fluff off her clothes. She was restless and frequently moved her position throughout interview. She talked rapidly in a soft voice although she became less nervous during interview and was fairly relaxed at the end. She appeared inhibited at talking about sexual difficulties and preferred talking at length about her phobic symptoms, which she insisted lay behind all her difficulties. *This is a correct interpretation. Once her phobic symptoms are treated she will feel more secure and her sexual difficulties will resolve.*

Formal Diagnosis: Agoraphobia

Treatment will consist of extinguishing the conditioned avoidance response by gradual exposure to the feared situations along the lines discussed earlier. Once this has been completed successfully no further treatment is needed as the normal pattern of behaviour should become self-reinforcing. The most convincing evidence that the behavioural model is appropriate for this type of patient is the favourable result of behaviour therapy (Marks, 1987). This has conclusively shown itself to be effective in phobic disorders and its success deals with all the objections raised by other models.

Our case history illustrates that the psychiatrist here is predominantly concerned with abnormal behaviour and although a full history with development and progression is taken there is no need for detailed enquiry about personal relationships and exploration of psychic conflict. The psychodynamic model regards the association of agoraphobic symptoms and frigidity as understandable as going out of doors and walking down the street is recognized by dream analysts to be symbolic of sexual intercourse. But this is irrelevant to the work of behaviour therapy and, if true, removal of the symptom will be ineffective.

Our phobic patient was treated by counter-conditioning but classical and operant conditioning were also used in treatment. Classical conditioning is best represented in the form of *aversion therapy*. For example, the continual excess of drinking of the alcoholic is maladaptive because it leads to further drinking and increased problems in living. Unfortunately the harm caused by alcohol abuse is delayed whilst its immediate effect is often pleasurable. It follows from the laws of conditioning that drinking behaviour therefore tends to be reinforced. The maladaptive response is 'alcohol (not just in the form of Guinness) is good for you', and solves many of life's problems. In aversion therapy a highly unpleasant negative stimulus–response pattern is placed as close as possible to the reinforcing maladaptive one in the expectation that the two will link together. If this happens the drinking of alcohol becomes associated with nasty feelings that overcome the former pleasurable ones.

In aversion therapy for alcohol abuse, vomiting is the most commonly induced negative response. An injection or drink of a drug which causes vomiting (apomorphine or emetine) is given and followed immediately by the consumption of alcohol. The unfortunate patient then passes through a cycle of retching, vomiting, giddiness and wretchedness. To add authenticity to the proceedings the drinking is staged in a congenial setting, with soft lights, music and general *bonhomie*. But as soon as the nausea and vomiting begins the attitudes of the staff change and the sufferer is berated for the squalor and degradation he has brought on himself, and which will continue as long as he goes on drinking. An outsider seeing this little drama might be excused for thinking that the treatment was sadistic and inhumane and its sole object was to humiliate the victim of the exercise. This immediate reaction is understandable but when it is realized that the alcoholic is an informed partner to the treatment and that the behaviour of the staff is designed to maximize the

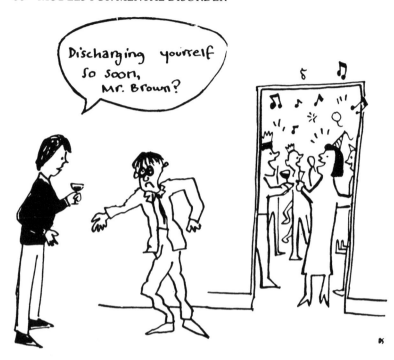

'To add authenticity to the proceedings . . .'

effects of negative reinforcement, ultimately for the patient's benefit, such criticism evaporates. The treatment can, in any case, be modified to avoid vomiting while still producing negative reinforcement (Blake, 1965).

The key question is, does the treatment work? One only needs to see people treated successfully by aversion techniques to be reassured of its value. A similar approach is to show a patient what he was like when inebriated. Amnesia is common among alcoholics and they remember little of their behaviour after prolonged drinking. By recording videotapes of behaviour after admission to hospital and showing these to the patient when sober a much better awareness of the effects of alcohol abuse is shown. The videotape is another negative reinforcer. Obviously the behaviourist is not just satisfied with removing a response pattern by negative means. He also wants to reinforce positively other adaptive patterns of behaviour. For example, if one of the initial reasons for drinking is the feeling of embarrassment with people a programme of *social skills training* leading to greater confidence in personal relationships and a lessened need for the apparent support of alcohol may be introduced.

Operant conditioning is also widely used with clinical problems. Abnormal behaviour in children can be treated and has been particularly successful in the training of mentally handicapped children. A behaviour such as feeding oneself without help is often a major hurdle for the handicapped child. In the past inability to carry out this (and similar behaviour which the intellectually normal child does not think twice about) was accepted as part and parcel of mental handicap. Now we realize that the potential to achieve greater independence is present in many of these children. Operant conditioning techniques can be employed, with successful feeding behaviour being rewarded and failed feeding ignored. This is not as easy as it sounds, for it is difficult not to give the incompetent child more attention than the successful one, and attention is a powerful reinforcer. In other types of abnormal behaviour, particularly those which are destructive and disruptive, stronger negative reinforcement may be used. An alternative, which is neither a positive nor a negative reinforcement consists of isolating the child for a short period. The reader may have come across the term *'time out'*, which describes this approach. It removes the child from an environment where reward is possible and can be much more helpful than punishments for behaviour disturbance, which may satisfy the child's need for attention although on the surface it appears to have no possible attractions.

A therapist well-trained in learning theory is able to design a programme for treating every sort of abnormal behaviour. The first part of assessment is to find out if there are any precipitants of the behaviour and whether it is predictable (*a behavioural or functional analysis*). Responses that lessen or increase the behaviour (positive and negative reinforcers) are then studied, and a good *behavioural modification programme* should have an approximately even number of these. The idea that behaviourists have a penchant to punish is a myth; they much prefer to reward. The programme is constructed and all personnel involved with the client, be they parents, children, nurses or doctors, are seen and agreement reached on the running of the programme. This is important because if there is inconsistency between the different personnel involved with treatment its effectiveness will be greatly reduced. As conditioning is so dependent on the interval between stimulus and response, adaptive or maladaptive behaviour should as far as possible be reinforced immediately. Treatment is concluded when all the abnormal behaviour is extinguished and a healthy pattern of response established. Occasionally 'booster doses' of treatment are required but as most normal responses are kept normal by the positive and negative reinforcement of healthy social environmental interaction, the normal responses usually persist without any further interference. Even more serious forms of apparent psychiatric illness have been treated by these techniques. The hallucinations and delusions of schizophrenia have been successfully controlled by behavioural methods, although these techniques are still in their infancy and not yet widely available. The whole gamut of psychiatric syndromes lies at the behaviourist's feet waiting to be treated by a scientifically designed treatment that is both theoretically sound and practically effective.

The critics dismiss these claims as grandiose and premature. The assertion that the symptoms are the illness is one that particularly aggravates the advocate of the psychodynamic model. What is shown as behaviour is only the end product of a complicated series of processes involving the conscious and unconscious mind. To claim that abnormal behaviour is synonymous with illness ignores all these factors. A man who intended to commit suicide, drives to a high cliff and then jumps to his death only shows abnormal behaviour in the last seconds of his life, but the mental processes that led to his suicide preceded the behaviour by many weeks or months. If the suicide leap was prevented by a temporary form of positive reinforcement it would only be repeated later in another form if the underlying conflict was not resolved. Behaviourism is just not enough to explain the creative genius of Beethoven, Shakespeare, Leonardo da Vinci and Michelangelo. It is laughable to pretend that their work was just the end product of conditioned and unconditioned reflexes, of well-positioned positive and negative reinforcement, otherwise we could all achieve the same powers.

The behaviourist acknowledges these attacks; he has heard them all before and is used to their emotional tone and rhetorical questions. His answer is that he is not issuing a prescription for the human condition, but is concerned simply with maladaptive functioning. He is concerned with the relief of abnormal patterns of behaviour, which unlike normal functioning, are relatively few and stereotyped. He replies to the Shavian criticism that all the principles of behaviour therapy are self-evident and require no special knowledge by pointing out that many common-sense ways of dealing with problems are inappropriate and lead to maladaptive learning. The mother who goes and cuddles her child every time she shows the slightest distress is very likely to set up an attention-seeking pattern of response. The child is rewarded by a cuddle whenever she is upset, so before long she learns to pretend to be upset whenever she wants her mother's attention. The man who burgles a house and is caught in the act does not get punished

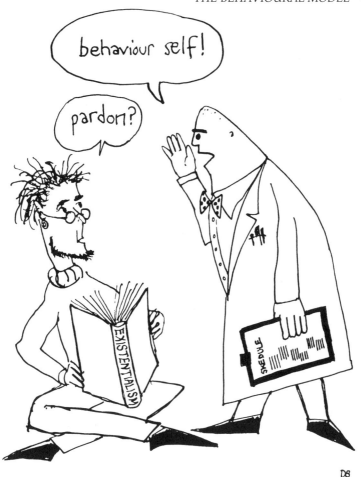

'It is laughable to pretend that their work was just the end product . . .'

immediately. He usually appears in court and is released on bail. Many weeks later he goes on trial and may go to prison. The negative reinforcement of imprisonment is far removed in time from the crime and we know from learning theory that any unconditioned response that develops will be a weak one. But what happens if the burglar is not caught? He gets a positive reinforcement immediately when he escapes with his loot. So it is hardly surprising that petty thieving becomes a career, and we breed recidivists, apparently incorrigible rogues who are 'incapable of learning right from wrong'. Of course they are quite capable of learning correctly but we would have to alter the system of reward and punishment for it to be effective.

The behaviourist can also show that to dismiss learning theory because it is based on a series of simple reflexes is premature. As behaviour therapy develops, more complex techniques are introduced which are far removed from simple Pavlovian conditioning. Modelling, of which mention has already been made, involves showing the ideal form of behaviour to a client (e.g. showing a film of a calm patient receiving dental treatment) and another, shaping, involves reinforcing successively closer approximations to the required response. However much we try to forget it, our complex and apparently original behaviour is composed of many smaller units of behaviour which obey certain established laws. This is no different from saying that deep down we all have the same basic structural unit, the double helix of the DNA molecule. Why no-one takes exception to this, yet waxes eloquently about the simplistic model of learning theory, is beyond the behaviourist's comprehension.

The behavioural model is also at odds with the disease model on many issues. It maintains that the sick role is inappropriate for many psychological disorders, and may contribute to handicap. Worse still, it may create new illness (i.e. is iatrogenic). By adopting a passive role the patient is rewarded by the medical model. Like a lump of clay on the potter's wheel he is moulded into a shape chosen by the doctor. This shape may be right or wholly inappropriate but it is more likely to be the latter, as the doctor is limited by his organic orientation and through his blinkered eyes can only recognize disease. Our clay patient is returned to society in his new mould only to return sharply when he realizes he still does not fit. So a cycle of admission and relapses follows (about half of all psychiatric in-patients are readmitted to hospital) until either the doctor or patient retires through exhaustion. What worries the behaviourist is that each time the patient adopts the sick role, whether it is appropriate or not, he is rewarded by attention by the prestigious medical profession.

If doctors were a profession provoking abuse and disdain the attention would not be rewarding, but as things stand at present all such attention positively reinforces the sick role. So the person, or client to the behaviourist, becomes a patient to the doctor. At subsequent consultation and relapses his power to shape his own destiny is gradually whittled away until he no longer thinks or acts independently, reaching its final form in the stereotyped institutional behaviour of the chronic hospitalized patient. This state has been reproduced in animals when they are placed in situations where others decide what happens to them. It is an apathetic, sad condition

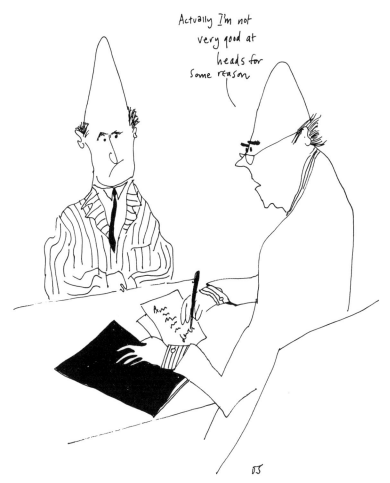

'This shape may be right or wholly inappropriate . . .'

which has been called learned helplessness. Doctors who follow the disease model unwittingly encourage helplessness and thereby promote new 'illness'.

The behaviourist has more sympathy with the cognitive model discussed in the next chapter. He nonetheless remains concerned that changing thinking does not automatically lead to a change in behaviour. He therefore prefers the cognitive element of treatment to be secondary to the behavioural one.

Behavioural treatment sets out clearly the roles of therapists and client, often in the form of a contract. Treatment contracts are a product of the behaviouristic approach and have now developed beyond the confines of learning theory. They establish the goals the client has to attain before improvement can be achieved or the next stage of treatment begun, and also demarcate the responsibilities of the therapist as well as the client.

The hierarchy of medicine is alien to the behavioural therapist. There is no need for an authoritarian approach in behaviour therapy. The person with the necessary skills is the one who organizes the treatment. Others in a team may be involved in carrying out the programme but a two-way contract between treaters and treated cannot develop in a hierarchical atmosphere. It is no good telling patients that a treatment is to be given because the expert has decided that this is the best available. No behavioural treatment will be effective unless the reasons for choosing it are explained and cooperation obtained. So it is in everyone's interests to have an informal relationship between the parties concerned and to avoid the pronouncements of authority. Moreover, the goals, methods and indeed the reasons of behaviour therapy can be readily discussed in plain language by therapist and patient.

The behaviourist is also able to dismiss another bogy that is frequently resurrected when behaviour therapy is being criticized, that of symptom substitution. This concept has developed from psychodynamic theory, particularly from the 'hydraulic' concepts of Freud. Symptoms, according to Freud, are the unhealthy expression of libidinous forces. These forces would be expressed differently if the ego and super-ego allowed them to come out into the open. Because they are repressed and denied they surface in an alien form, psychiatric symptoms, which are acceptable to the ego because they completely disguise the real problem. It therefore follows that if these symptoms are merely regarded as the illness in its entirety, and treatment focused only on removing them, that the problem is going to resurface in another form. Like the hydra of Greek mythology, if one head is chopped off two new ones will grow in its place. So new symptoms will be substituted for old ones and until the therapist explores more deeply no real progress will be made.

The behaviourist notes this theoretical criticism. Instead of responding in kind with an equally plausible defence of symptomatic treatment he turns to the empirical evidence. When follow-up studies of behaviour therapy are examined there is no evidence that symptom substitution occurs to any appreciable extent. If there is a return of symptoms it is almost always of the same nature as the original symptoms. Symptoms substitution as a criticism of behaviour therapy collapses under the weight of this evidence and should not inhibit the behaviour therapist.

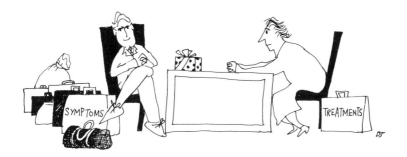

'So new symptoms will be substituted for old ones . . .'

The advocates of the social model are also unhappy about the spread of behaviour therapy, but for different reasons. The concept of conditioning and reflex control worries them because although they may at first be used to remove unpleasant symptoms it is easy to abuse them and use them to induce conformity. For example, homosexuality was formerly considered a criminal offence but in our more enlightened times is usually accepted as part of the range of normal behaviour. Behaviour therapy has helped to promote this change but may have led to attitudes that homosexuality is a form of abnormal behaviour that needs to be extinguished. The behavioural treatment of homosexuality regards it in exactly this way. In its simplest form the client is negatively reinforced (e.g. by receiving an electric shock) whenever he shows a sexual response (e.g. engorgement of the penis recorded by a blood flow measurement called penile plethysmography) to a nude photograph of a member of his own sex and positively reinforced by similar responses to the opposite sex. The homosexual response is therefore treated as deviant and unhealthy. The techniques of brainwashing have been developed along the same lines and people can be forced to believe things and behave in ways that are entirely alien to them. However, this sort of argument follows from the effectiveness of behaviour therapy, not its supposed moral or political position. If someone wished to change his sexual orientation, or any other preference, behaviour therapy offers an effective, voluntary means of doing so.

The behaviourist is aware of the powers that his treatment possesses but can claim with justification that although all successful therapies can be abused this is not a reason for abandoning them. He can also emphasize that in the therapeutic use of behaviour therapy the patient should be motivated to come for treatment and not be dragooned by an external agency. This is not just pious talk, because those who come for behaviour therapy against their will, be they homosexual, phobic or obsessional, will show little or no response. It is only in a society entirely ruled by Orwellian conformity that brainwashing would be commonplace and it is up to us as political beings to ensure that such a society never develops. But it would be quite wrong to deprive psychology of an effective treatment because of this potential danger.

The behaviour model brings psychiatric disorders out from the murky caves of dynamic theory and examines them in the light of day. It records and treats what it observes, and scorns conjecture. Most psychiatric disorder is grist to its mill because it consists of abnormal behaviour rather than disease. It has a firm scientific base in experimental psychology and this enables it to plan and predict the effects of treatment instead of relying on empiricism alone. Although it is a relatively recent newcomer to psychiatry its supporters are confident it will become the major impetus for progress in the future. Tomrrow's students of psychiatry will need to know much more of learning theory and less of the minutiae of disease if they are to become effective practitioners, and despite its adaptability and sophistication its principles are logical and straightforward.

REFERENCES

Blake, B.G. (1965) The application of behaviour therapy to the treatment of alcoholism. *Behaviour Research and Therapy*, **3**, 75–80.

Marks, I.M. (1987) *Fears, Phobias and Rituals: Panic, Anxiety and Their Disorders*. Oxford University Press, London.

Orwell, G. (1949) *1984*. Secker and Warburg, London.

Pavlov, I.P. (1927) *Conditioned Reflexes*. Oxford University Press, London.

Pavlov, I.P. (1941) *Conditioned Reflexes and Psychiatry*. International Publishers, New York.

Shaw, G.B. (1932) *The Adventures of the Black Girl in Her Search for God*. Constable and Co, London.

Skinner, B.F. (1972) *Beyond freedom and dignity*. Jonathan Cape, London.

Watson, J.B. and Rayner, R. (1920) Conditioned emotional reactions. *Journal of Experimental Psychology*, **3**, 1–14.

Wolpe, J. (1958) *Psychotherapy by reciprocal inhibition*. Stanford University Press, Stanford.

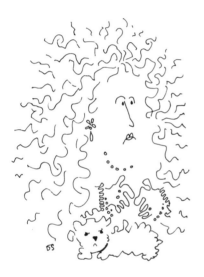

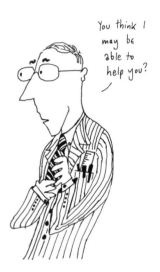

'. . . errors or biases in thinking'

CHAPTER 5

The Cognitive Model

'And thus the native hue of resolution
Is sicklied o'er with the pale cast of thought'
William Shakespeare, *Hamlet*

This is a new model that has achieved great strides in the 20 years since it was first formulated. Like many models in psychiatry it began as a form of treatment, primarily for depression and anxiety (Beck 1976, Beck *et al.* 1985, Blackburn & Davidson 1990) but now has been extended to cover almost all of psychiatry. The basic tenet of the model is simple: much of mental disorder is created by errors or biases in thinking. The thinking of society and therapists may be at fault, but that is not the important issue. It is the dysfunctional thinking of the patient in response to a variety of stimuli that creates mental disorder that would not otherwise be present.

At first sight this is a curious notion. Are other proponents of the cognitive model suggesting the mental disorder is 'all in the mind'? Surely thinking becomes disordered as a consequence of illness; can it really be the primary cause?

To answer these questions let us take a common superstition of childhood, touching a lamp-post before crossing the road. There are many childhood superstitions of this nature, including those about numbers and days (e.g. only having a bath on a Thursday), walking on pavements (walking only on the lines or in the squares) or counting to a certain number on your fingers before undertaking an important task (e.g. running in a school race). In the case of touching the lamp-post before crossing the road it is easy to see how the symptom could arise. The child is taught by his mother to be careful when crossing roads and, early in his life, he always has to cross

77

accompanied. He recognizes that this activity is associated with some danger and so care needs to be exercised when crossing roads. Touching a lamp-post before crossing can give an irrational sense of security; the child feels that in some magical way he is protected from danger when he crosses.

The behaviourist regards the act of touching the lamp-post as the important component of this sequence. If there is no lamp-post to touch and the child becomes agitated and anxious, and will have to make a detour to cross the road at another point, then behavioural methods will be needed to treat what has become a disorder. However, the prime mover in this sequence is the superstitious thought, not the behaviour. If we can persuade the young boy that there is no rational need to touch a lamp-post before crossing a road and that it would be much more sensible to follow the highway code to ensure a road is safe to cross, then one (slightly) maladaptive behaviour is followed by an adaptive one.

This problem, described in this way, is not yet severe enough to be a psychiatric disorder but it can easily become so if the child's thinking about the problem remains distorted. A whole series of persistent repetitive thoughts (ruminations) or actions (rituals) can develop to avoid a host of imaginary dangers, not just when crossing roads but in every part of life. More and more time is spent in these unnecessary activities (which now are severe enough to be called obsessional symptoms) and they prevent normal functioning. In extreme cases the person can be totally crippled by these symptoms so that no useful activity is carried out. Again the behaviourist regards the prime problem as the abnormal repetitive useless acts, but these are not carried out in isolation; if the person did not think they served some protective functioning (usually for the relief of anxiety) there would be no need to carry them out.

To examine the value of the cognitive model let us look at a typical problem where treatment related to the model, cognitive therapy, is used as the main line of treatment.

CASE HISTORY

Presenting Problem

A 29-year-old woman was referred to the psychiatrist by the general practitioner because of recurrent anxiety amd depressive symptoms complicated by concerns about her health. Part of his letter read: 'she often calls me out in the evening or presents to the casualty department in the middle of the night, convinced she is having a heart attack, and although I have reassured her that all the tests are normal and she has no evidence of any heart disease she does not believe me. I am frustrated with her and she is frustrated with me. She has become more depressed recently and says that she cannot go on feeling like this. I am particularly concerned now because she has threatened suicide if there is no hope of an end to her troubles'.

When seen the woman explained that she had been quite well until nine months previously. She then had an acute attack of palpitations and sweating while resting quietly at home after a busy day. During this attack she was convinced she would pass out and thought that she might be having a heart attack. She called her doctor, who came to see her within half an hour, examined her and could find nothing wrong. By this time she had recovered from her attack and was not surprised that the doctor found nothing of significance, and so she responded to his reassurance. Four days later she had another attack while sitting at a word processor at her work at a bank where she was a senior secretary. She had the same palpitations and sweating and when, after about five minutes, she started feeling that she was going to collapse she was again convinced that her doctor must have been wrong and she was having a heart attack. Her work colleagues saw her in this state and agreed that there must be something seriously wrong. An occupational health nurse saw her immediately and rushed her to a local casualty department. She was examined fully by several doctors in the department and had a range of further tests, including electrocardiograms. A systolic murmur was noted and she was advised to come back for further tests at a cardiology clinic.

Subsequently, however, these tests confirmed no significant cardiac pathology and she was again reassured. By this time she was convinced that the doctors must be wrong because she was continuing to have these attacks and they were occurring up to four times a week. She could never predict when they would occur and was angry when her general practitioner suggested they might be related to stress. She described clearly that they occurred unpredictably in many situations, often when she was sitting relaxed in a chair. More recently she had also developed pain in the lower ribs and this, in her mind, confirmed that she was likely to be suffering from a heart condition.

Her general practitioner suggested referring her to his practice nurse for counselling, but this was rejected angrily by the patient who insisted that her problem was not a psychological one. However, as her attacks continued she became her more demoralized and depressed. She could see no future, and at times did not mind if she died in one of her attacks as at least this would 'solve the problem'. She saw no point in living while her attacks continued and later developed feelings of guilt about consulting her general practitioner so frequently. When she said to him that she was becoming a burden on his practice and might it not be better if she were dead the general practitioner became alarmed and persuaded her to be referred to the psychiatrist.

Assessment and Treatment

The psychiatrist, who was also a cognitive therapist, noted that the patient was obviously depressed at interview. She looked unhappy, frequently apologized for wasting his time and said that nobody wanted to help her anyway as she was not worth helping. The conversation continued:-

Psychiatrist: If you aren't worth helping why do you think your doctor referred you to the clinic?

Patient: He just wanted to get me off his hands. My friends are the same. They don't want to talk to me any more; I'm such a pain. They just want me to disappear from their lives.

Psychiatrist: What evidence do you have for these thoughts?

Patient: Because they stay out of my way. They avoid talking to me unless they have to. Talking to me is just like a duty for them.

Psychiatrist: Doesn't anybody care about you?

Patient: No, I'm sure they don't.

Psychiatrist: So one possibility is that no one cares but another is that they do still care about you? Do they still come and see you?

Patient: Yes. My best friend came last week but talking to her made no difference so I told her to go away.

Psychiatrist: So your friends keep on coming even though you tell them to go away. That seems an odd sort of thing to do if they don't care about you.

Patient: I don't think they really care. They just feel it's their duty to come and see me.

Psychiatrist: How else could they prove they care except by coming to see you?

Patient: I don't know.

Psychiatrist: If you were in their position how would you show that you cared?

Patient: I suppose I'd keep on coming like they do and try to cheer me up.

Psychiatrist: So it is possible they do care about you and are trying to help as best they can?

Patient: I suppose so.

If you look at this conversation again closely you will see that the patient has a pattern of thinking that does not fit in with the facts. She assumes that nobody cares about her although there is some evidence to the contrary. For the adherents of the disease model, these depressive thoughts are a direct consequence of the biochemical disturbance lying behind depressive illness. For the cognitive therapist, however, these thoughts lead to increasing levels of depression, or, more commonly, its perpetuation and development. Rather than contradicting the patient, the therapist explores what has actually been happening and thereby directly challenges the patient's assumption that she is disliked and ignored. This is an essential part of cognitive therapy, nicely summed up as *collaborative empiricism*, the therapist exploring the patient's thinking patterns and gently illustrating that there are alternative more appropriate and adaptive thoughts that could equally well be possessed by the patient.

In further discussions the patient repeated the same negative line of thinking when describing her doctor's attitude. She had interpreted his comments that there was nothing seriously wrong with her physical health as a direct contradiction of her own feelings. 'He kept saying there was nothing wrong' she said, 'but I knew the way I felt. I was having these attacks when I felt awful and never had them before, so obviously something was wrong.' She had gone further in her depressive thinking by interpreting the doctor's reassurance about her physical health as a wish to dismiss her from the surgery as she was becoming a nuisance. First she blamed the doctor for what she construed as misdiagnosis, but later she blamed herself (One of the reasons for this is that as she became more depressed her panic attacks disappeared. She therefore thought that perhaps her symptoms during these attacks might have been less 'real' than she at first thought and that perhaps she was to blame for bothering the doctor.)

After the end of the first session of treatment the patient was asked to keep a diary of the time she felt particularly depressed or particularly anxious and nervous over the week before her next appointment. On each occasion she felt either depressed or nervous she was asked to rate her feelings on a scale between 0 and 10 (more severe symptoms scoring higher), and also asked to record what she was thinking at the time she felt this way. The need for this 'homework' was explained by the therapist and the need to have a verbatim account of each of these episodes together with the thinking at the time, not a reconstruction of the thinking that almost certainly would have intruded if the patient had waited until the next appointment before describing these feelings. In subsequent treatment sessions the patient was able to identify that she felt most depressed when she was alone and most cheerful when she was with her friends or acquaintances.

After three further sessions she was much less depressed and, although she still had times when she had a negative self-image and wanted to shut herself away from people, she was no longer despairing. As she put it, 'I've got my thinking under control now. The depression doesn't just arrive and take over; I can get rid of it when I want'.

Subsequently, and which sometimes happens in clinical practice when depression is relieved, she became more anxious again and had further panic attacks. The therapist was able to explain the symptoms from knowledge of basic physiology so that she realized that although they were real they could be explained without recourse to a disease explanation. The continuing of homework diaries established that her panic attacks were not entirely unpredictable as they all occurred at the end of the day and were much more frequent when she was under additional pressure at work. She recognized this link and altered her work to reduce this stress. Again in explaining her symptoms on subsequent appointments she emphasized that she was now in control of these feelings and they no longer dominated her life as they had done previously.

FUNDAMENTALS OF THE COGNITIVE MODEL

The treatment of this woman demonstrates that she has a number of abnormal thoughts and that these are not secondary features. The term 'dysfunctional' is often used to describe them, and although this is an unwieldy adjective, it is an accurate one; these thoughts impair healthy function. By directly changing them the clinical picture changes completely and she improves. This is not just an artificial textbook case. This improvement is common in treatment and close examination of the changes that occur before improvement reveals why.

Firstly it was necessary to deal with the (secondary) depressive symptoms that were handicapping progress in treating her anxiety attacks. At one level it is easy to see why she became demoralized because no one was giving her an adequate explanation of her attacks. She was getting negative information that there was nothing seriously wrong, but this was not replaced by new insights into possible causes and explanations for her symptoms. However, her subsequent reaction, to withdraw from contact with her friends, to feel that nothing would ever improve and that she would be better off dead, was clearly pathological.

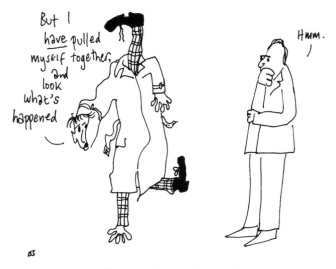

'. . . pull yourself together . . .'

The common-sense approach to these feelings is along the lines of 'don't be silly, pull yourself together and don't go on thinking like this'. This approach, although derided, can be of some benefit, but not when these thoughts have become established firmly.

You will note from the progress of treatment that the therapist does not get involved in an argument with the patient about correct and incorrect thoughts. Instead there is a 'twin track' approach whereby the therapist aligns with the patient's thinking and analyses these thoughts in a rational manner. This is illustrated in Table 5.1 and the process is seen to work specifically for the patient's symptoms of depression and, later, for the symptoms of panic, because after analysis these are seen by the patient to be those of panic rather than those of physical disease. It will be noted that the therapist does not immediately jump to the conclusion that these are panic attacks because this implies a psychological cause; instead the patient comes to this conclusion for herself and as a result its impact is much greater and the inappropriate thoughts are replaced by rational ones. By the end of therapy the patient's thinking has become more adaptive and the symptoms, no longer reinforced by abnormal thoughts, fade away because they have ceased to be of any importance.

The cognitive model not only emphasizes the role of abnormal thoughts in both creating and maintaining abnormal mental states but also helps to give the patient the sense of mastery over feelings that were previously beyond voluntary control. This is of immense therapeutic benefit. Just imagine if you had a severe attack of panic

Table 5.1   Twin-track thinking in cognitive therapy

Patient's thoughts	Therapist's thoughts and responses
I am useless, no one cares about me	She is pushing people away and then blames them for not seeing her *Response:* find out who is seeing her and test if she feels they really do not care
No one believes anything I say	She will not entertain any explanations for her condition that conflict with her own views *Response:* test if she really means that no one reinforces her views
It's a waste of time people talking to me	She does not listen properly to other people *Response:* is that the view of others too? Why do they still come and see you?
People only come to see me out of a sense of duty	We are making progress; she is thinking of others' reactions *Response:* how do you know? Put yourself in their position, how would you react?
I feel faint and have palpitations, therefore I am having a heart attack	She is misinterpreting symptoms of anxiety. *Response:* Could there be other explanations that are at least equally tenable?
I suppose so. I'm still here and the doctors cannot find anything wrong	Possibility of anxiety as a cause can be introduced *Response:* It is possible to feel this way when you are under a lot of stress
I suppose I ought to look seriously at the possibility that these feelings are due to stress in my life	

while reading these words. We presume you will be reading them in the fairly neutral environment which is not particularly threatening. You suddenly develop difficulty in breathing, palpitations, a cold sweat and a feeling of impending catastrophe. You try and work out what is going on but cannot find an explanation. Your body seems to be crying out in terror but there is nothing to be frightened of. Is it really surprising that under these circumstances you will come to the conclusion that there is some major abnormality of your body's function that can only be explained by a serious disease?

Now consider how your reaction would be if you had received successful cognitive therapy. You notice the symptoms of difficulty in breathing and palpitations, as before. You immediately recognize them as being part of the panic attack which will do you no physical harm. Consciously, or sometimes automatically without really thinking about it, you breath a little more slowly and deeply and find yourself relaxing. The feeling of panic goes away, partly because you have become less anxious as the panic has not reinforced itself like a vicious dragon chasing its own tail, but also because you *know* how to deal with these symptoms when they arise. When these feelings no longer descend on you like some sort of alien force that you can do nothing about and instead you have regarded it as part and parcel of your body's own reactions that you can control, then they no longer pose any real threat. You are in control of them.

THE COGNITIVE MODEL IN OTHER MENTAL DISORDERS

So far we have described the application of the cognitive model to depressive, anxiety and hypochondriacal symptoms. The model could also be applied to many other conditions, including eating disorders (Freeman *et al.*, 1988), personality disorder (Beck, 1991), alcohol and drug abuse, disorders of sleep and other problems of physiological functions, and marital disorders (Schmaling *et al.*, 1989). The approach will be evident from the general principles of the model. Thus the central preoccupation of the anorexic girl that her body is obscenely fat, the patient with the personality disorder whose close relationships keep on breaking down but in every case he is not responsible for this, the alcoholic who thinks that whenever he feels depressed alcohol will cheer him up, and the insomniac who feels that he never sleeps a wink and will die from perpetual wakefulness, all have similar dysfunctional thoughts. The adaptive, appropriate, rational thoughts are not easy to substitute for the irrational ones, but it can be done by a collaborative, empirical approach of cognitive therapy.

A useful analogy is to think of a team of horses pulling a coach. Normally the coachman is in control and the horses stay still, trot or gallop at the coachman's command. But in these disorders the horses are out of control; the coachman can do nothing except warn the passengers to take evading action and hope that the horses will come to their senses before they or the people on the coach suffer serious injury. The response to the reins is irrational and so irrationality reigns.

The cognitive therapist is represented by the rider who gallops alongside the horses, calms them down so that eventually they stop or, if this does not work, leaves his own mount and jumps astride one of the lead horses and calms down the frightened animal gradually. 'This behaviour is irrational' is the message communicated to the horses, 'think about it a little and you'll find a better way.'

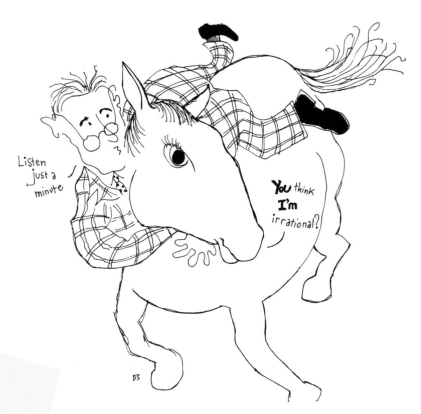

It could be argued that cognitive models do not apply to some other more serious mental disorders, particularly schizophrenia. Even in this group of conditions, however, abnormal cognitions are not necessarily beyond the reach of the cognitive approach (Kingdon & Turkington, 1993). Many patients with these disorders are able to recognize that their thoughts are abnormal and lead to beliefs that cannot be sustained. In the language of conventional psychiatry they have partial insight. There are also encouraging reports that these patients can replace dysfunctional thoughts (e.g. 'I think that those people standing on the other side of the street talking to each other are plotting to kill me' with more appropriate ones, 'although I sometimes think that people such as those standing across the street are plotting against me they could be talking about something completely different and I must not always jump to conclusions').

SUMMARY

The cognitive model is young and thriving and has far to go. It focuses on those faculties that make *Homo sapiens* different from all other animal species; we interpret our thoughts and they are the main determinants of our actions. Cognitive therapy shows that amazing versatility of the human mind; we can use our thinking processes to alter our view of ourselves, our worlds and the future. These are not the vague, inchoate thoughts addressed in psychodynamic theory or the phenomenological niceties of the disease model of psychiatry, but the important unadulterated thoughts that determine our day-to-day actions. Unlike the behavioural model, which alters behaviour first and ignores its precursors, the cognitive model aims to alter the thoughts that determine that behaviour. The two are not usually antagonistic, and indeed there is a growing discipline of cognitive behavioural therapy. For the cognitive theorist argues with conviction that although actions speak louder than words, thoughts speak louder and longer than actions.

REFERENCES

Beck, A.T. (1976) *Cognitive Therapy and the Emotional Disorders.* International Universities Press, New York.

Beck, A.T. (1991) *Cognitive Therapy of Personality Disorders.* Guilford Press, New York and London.

Beck, A.T., Emery, G. and Greenberg, R. (1985) *Anxiety Disorders and Phobias: a Cognitive Perspective.* Basic Books, New York.

Blackburn, I.M. and Davidson, K.M. (1990) *Cognitive Therapy in Depression and Anxiety.* Blackwell Scientific Publications, Oxford.

Freeman, C.P., Barry, F., *et al.* (1988) Controlled trial of psychotherapy for bulimia nervosa. *British Medical Journal,* **296**, 521–525.

Kingdon, D. and Turkington, D. (1993) *Cognitive Therapy in Schizophrenia.* Guilford Press, New York.

Schmaling, K.B., Fruzzetti, A.E. and Jacobson, N.S. (1989) Marital problems. In *Cognitive Behaviour Therapy for Psychiatric Problems,* (ed) K. Hawton, P. Salkovskis, J. Kirk and D.M. Clark, pp. 339–369. Oxford Medical, Oxford.

FURTHER READING

Ellis, A. (1962) *Reason and Emotion in Psychotherapy.* Stuart, New York.

Guidano, V.F. and Liotti, G. (1983) *Cognitive Processes and Emotional Disorders: a Structural Approach to Psychotherapy.* Guilford Press, New York and London.

Hawton, K., Salkovskis, P.M. *et al.* (eds) (1989) *Cognitive Behaviour Therapy for Psychiatric Problems: a Practical Guide.* Oxford Medical, Oxford.

CHAPTER 6

The Social Model

'We do not look out for any particular organ as the seat of insanity, nor do we pretend to operate directly on the mind or soul, but we aim to study the patient as a unity, as an individuum in all his physical, intellectual, moral and social relations.'

H van Leeuwen (Dutch psychiatrist), 1854

All social models in psychiatry have the same fundamental premise. They regard the wider influence of social forces as more important than other influences as causes or precipitants of mental illness. At a superficial level the social model appears to be a simple extension of the psychodynamic model. Whereas the dynamic model sees the patient in the context of his personal relationships, particularly those within the family, the social model sees him as a player on a much larger stage, that of society as a whole. But this implies that the methods of the psychodynamic model will be equally appropriate for the social one. This is not true as there are other important differences between the models that are summarized in Table 6.1 and explored in more detail below.

Sociology and psychiatry have long enjoyed healthy collaboration, and the social psychiatry model of mental illness has developed from this. Perhaps Emil Durkheim should be regarded as the founding member of the social psychiatry school. In his classical work on suicide in 1897 he showed that social factors, particularly isolation and its accompanying loss of social bonds, were important in predicting suicide and, indeed, in many instances appeared to be direct causes. The realization that mental illness was a direct consequence of social forces took time to take root as most psychiatrists of the day were followers of Kraepelin (disease model) or Freud

Table 6.1 Main differences between social and psychodynamic models

Causes of Disorder	
Psychodynamic model	Social model
Personal, highly specific, and not immediately understandable	Based on general theories of groups, communities and cultures
Unconscious mental mechanisms important in cause of mental illness	Observed environmental factors explain mental illness (e.g. social and economic pressures)
Past childhood conflicts explain present problems	Current or recently experienced conflicts explain problems
Symptoms determined by symbolic significance	Symptoms determined by nature of social event
Treated by personal or group psychotherapy	Treated by social and environmental changes

(psychodynamic model). The disease model was convinced that a physical explanation of psychiatric illness was just around the corner, and the psychodynamic model was busy looking beyond the obvious to the obscure. In the past 30 years the shortcomings of the other models have led to serious consideration and acceptance of the social model. Evidence for social forces being primary in the aetiology of much psychiatric illness is increasing (e.g. Totman 1979) and now the social model can stand unsupported.

In some ways it is surprising that it has taken so long for the social model to reach respectability in psychiatry. For years man has looked on many forms of illness as reactions to external events. People have been said to die 'from a broken heart' following the loss of a spouse for centuries; only recently has this been shown to have a scientific basis. After bereavement there is a higher risk of death in a spouse in the succeeding six months and heart disease is the commonest cause of death in this time (Parkes et al. 1967).

Where social psychologists and psychiatrists have made particular advances recently is in measuring the impact of social forces using acceptable scientific criteria. We know there are many social forces that can impinge on an individual but they vary greatly in degree and nature, and some may be a consequence rather than a cause of illness. Merely describing them is not enough for hypotheses to be tested; they have to be quantified. Holmes and Rahe were the first to introduce the concept of scaling life events. Their scale is called the Social Readjustment Rating Scale (Holmes & Rahe 1967), and there have been many others published since (e.g. Paykel et al. 1971). Holmes and Rahe quantified the severity of a particular life event by the degree of change it produces, and all events were recorded as life change units (LCU). The relative values of LCUs were determined by giving the scale of 42 items to 400 healthy people and asking them to record the amount of readjustment that each event would require. Although this may seem an idiosyncratic personal view a surprising degree of agreement was reached. All events carry an LCU score. An event such as bereavement scores 100 LCUs and one such as moving house scores only 20 LCUs. Further development of this and similar scales has separated events which are independent of illness from those which might be associated with it. For example, a person with an attack of bronchitis would often feel ill for a few days before developing chest symptoms and therefore not go to work. This does not mean that failure to go to work is a social cause of bronchitis. On the other hand, if a person gets abnormally depressed two weeks after his house is burgled, it is likely that the burglary was an important factor in the development of his depression as it is an independent event.

To varying degrees, life events have been shown to be important in the causation of mental illness. They are extremely important in neurotic disorders. It has been shown that such events are seven times greater in patients with these disorders than in matched control subjects (Cooper & Sylph 1973). This perhaps is so well known that it does not need repeating. Major upheavals in our lives are stressful and stress and mental illness often go together. The anxiety of the newly appointed business executive trying to keep to the schedules demanded by his company, the depression of a mother with young children who is deserted by her husband, the hypochondirasis of the nuclear power worker exposed to radiation, the impotence of a young man immediately following his marriage; they are all neurotic reactions which are immediately understandable in the context of life events and it would be foolish to consider

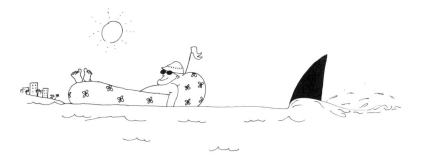

'We are all prone to mental disturbance when unpleasant events strike us without warning . . .'

the problems in isolation. We are all prone to mental disturbance when unpleasant events strike us without warning and 'stress reactions' are the most common mental disorders.

More severe mental illness used to be thought of in a different light. The adjective 'endogenous' is commonly used to indicate that such illness is independent of external 'exogenous' circumstances. It is as though there was an internal clock within the individual which predetermined when the episode of illness would start and the timing could not be altered in any way. We know this to be wrong. Schizophrenia, for example, used to be thought of as an illness that was independent of social factors. Its original name, dementia praecox (precocious dementia), illustrates this. But there is now abundant evidence that there are significantly more independent life events immediately before the onset of schizophrenia compared with a control population (Brown & Birley 1968) and that future relapse is not only dependent on life events (Vaughn & Leff 1973), but also on the level of emotion expressed by others that the patient experiences after leaving hospital. If there is a high level of critical emotion expressed then the patient is much more likely to relapse than if he is exposed to a calmer emotional context. It may therefore be preferable for a schizophrenic patient to return to a place that is relatively underestimated (e.g. a lodging house) after leaving hospital, instead of to the bosom of his family, where he may not be able to cope with the emotional pressures. There are also more life events immediately before the onset of severe depression (Paykel et al. 1969) and mania (Ambelas 1979), conditions which in the past were also thought to be 'endogenous'.

Recent work on depressed patients has shown that certain social factors are commonly found in such patients. Women living in a London borough were chosen at random and interviewed using a diagnostic schedule. The group diagnosed as depressed were found to have more young children at home, less full-time or part-time employment, and fewer confidants with whom to discuss their worries than the non-depressed group (Brown & Harris 1978). An interesting difference was found between the social factors in 'neurotic' and 'endogenous' depression. The time between major life changes (particularly those involving loss) and the depression was significantly greater for 'endogenously' depressed patients. Thus the apparently unpredictable onset of endogenous depression may be misleading; social factors are important but because those responsible may have been experienced many months or years before the depression begins they are missed. The interval between the onset of the precipitating social factors and the depression alters the form of the eventual illness so the clinical features of 'endogenous' and 'neurotic' depression differ.

IDENTIFICATION OF SOCIAL CAUSES OF MENTAL ILLNESS

It is not particularly difficult to identify the social factors that are responsible for mental illness. In fact, it is almost too easy, because the causes are so prominent that they are ignored by the investigator who tries to be too clever. For example, studies of alcoholism (now euphemistically called drinking problems) were carried out many years ago to determine the type of person most at risk. Many thought that the alcoholic was born with an abnormal form of metabolism that led to a greater risk of addiction. It is now known that the obvious precipitating factors, the availability and price of alcoholic drinks, are also the main causes of alcoholism. In countries where the price of alcohol is very high or the outlets to the public are strictly controlled there is a significantly lower incidence of alcoholism than in other countries, such as France and Italy, in which regular alcohol consumption is part of daily life.

As with the previous two models it is worth while studying a problem commonly seen in clinical practice to illustrate the value of the social model. The patient is a young man aged 24 who was first seen in a general hospital following a suicide attempt. He had taken an overdose of sleeping tablets after a fairly trivial row with his girlfriend. He is referred to the psychiatrist because he repeatedly expresses the view that life is hopeless and that there is nothing to live for. After questioning the young man about the reasons for the overdose it is clear to the doctor that there are many reasons for the patient to feel depressed and these cannot be regarded as personal matters that are in some ways under his control. He was made redundant from his job as an engineer 18 months ago and has not been able to get work since. This has been very disillusioning for him as he trained for three years as an engineering apprentice before taking up his job and thought that with this training he would have a job for life. Unfortunately, his company had shifted its interest towards microcomputers and no longer needed his skills.

He was now living on unemployment benefit which was less than half his original wage. With this income he was unable to save any money and was not able to obtain a mortgage to buy a house. He had hoped to raise sufficient cash for a down payment on a house before getting married but now his relationship with his girlfriend has begun to deteriorate. They were having repeated arguments, mainly about money, and on the night of the overdose she had threatened to leave him. *The young man has suffered two important losses for which he could not be held responsible. He has suffered loss of income because he was made redundant and loss of self-respect because he does not see himself as a useful member of society. No wonder he feels depressed.*

RELATIONSHIP BETWEEN CAUSES AND SYMPTOMS OF MENTAL ILLNESS

The psychodynamic model emphasizes that symptoms are not what they seem and serve as a means of distracting the therapist from the real cause of mental conflict. The social model maintains that mental illness is related clearly to social factors and there is no difficulty in predicting that one will follow from the other. For example, it has been shown in many studies that people who live in poor, deprived geographical areas, who are unemployed and in unsatisfactory housing and have no special occupational skills, are all likely to suffer higher rates of mental illness than the rest of the population. Throughout the Western world, mental health services for the inner cities have to cope with dramatically higher rates of referral than more affluent areas. It is therefore reasonable to conclude that these social circumstances are a major cause of mental illness.

It is also useful to look further and see whether the causes have any links with certain types of mental disorder. In general these links are present. For example, it has been shown that depression is not just related to additional life events but is especially associated with events that are constructed as loss. This can be the loss of a close relative or another person, of material possessions such as a house or car, or something more abstract such as an ideal, ambition or belief. Thus depression is preceded by many more 'exit' events than 'entrance' ones (Paykel *et al.* 1969). Similarly, there is evidence that anxiety, which is essentially a symptom implying threat or danger, is more likely to be preceded by events signifying danger or threat than depressive symptoms, and that mixed feelings of anxiety and depression are associated with mixed events signifying threat and loss (Finlay-Jones & Brown 1981).

To return to the case of the young man who has taken an overdose, it is easy to see the relationship between the cause and symptoms of his depression. Until recently he was making good progress in his job and had a settled future. Since then he has lost his job, has been unable to raise sufficient money as a down payment on his house, and on the night of the overdose was threatened with an even greater loss, that of his girlfriend. In telling the psychiatrist about his feelings he comes back repeatedly to the notion that he has given up trying to solve his problems. He maintains that all his attempts to overcome his employment, financial and personal problems are doomed to fail as each solution seems to be replaced by a greater problem. *This phenomenon of 'giving up' often marks the dividing line between illness and health. An important part of treatment will be to help him find alternative ways of recovering his self-esteem.*

The reader will see that there is a much simpler relationship between the causes and symptoms in the social model compared with the psychodynamic model. According to the psychotherapist most symptoms are false clues and only explained through symbolism, but in the social model they are directly related, and easily seen to be related, to the cause of the symptoms. They are also more closely related in time than with the psychodynamic model. The causes of the symptoms are usually to be found within the recent past with the social model whereas one invokes unconscious conflict in childhood more frequently in the dynamic model.

Because the social model sees the individual in the setting of society it does not have fixed ideas of what constitutes psychiatric illness. The disease, psychodynamic and behavioural models all look to an internal explanation of psychiatric illness that stands on its own. The social model is concerned that the labelling of psychiatric illness may create its own disorder, as once labelled as ill a person may feel he has to act the part. There is a view, exemplified in its most exaggerated form by the writings of Thomas Szasz (1961) that mental illness is not real illness but only a label that doctors place on patients when they deviate from the norm. It is perfectly legitimate for a patient to consult the doctor for help if he or she feels unwell but it is inappropriate for the doctor to act on behalf of society and give any form of treatment against the person's will. Because there are no objective tests for mental illness the doctor has no authority to carry out this type of treatment and it only succeeds in practice because the doctor and patient play their respective roles with enthusiasm.

Although Szasz's view goes rather further than most advocates of the social model, it demonstrates the importance of society in determining attitudes and opinions about mental illness. In general, illness is only thought to be present if the individual goes beyond the bounds of socially acceptable behaviour. A villager on the shores of Lake Mweru in the north of Zambia will consult his nearest nganga (tribal witch doctor) when he develops the belief that other people are interfering with his mind and persecuting him. With this type of mental disorder it is common for the nganga to organize a ceremony in which he wears native headdress and will command the evil spirits to depart from the patient's body and cease to torment him. Sometimes this may need to involve a whole community because without the remainder of the tribe being present, there is a danger that the evil spirits may descend on another member.

This type of ceremony is not far removed from a social gathering where everyone knows his role and duties and many have a good time. The patient is regarded as an unfortunate victim rather than a patient; the evil spirits have chosen to descent on him but they could have come equally to someone else.

Contrast this with a similar problem in a Western affluent society. The young man will interpret his symptoms differently because of his cultural background. He is more likely to complain that his mind has been taken over by spacemen from another planet. They control his thoughts and movements and instruct him what to do. When he complains about these symptoms he is recognized by his family and the rest of society as ill and medical help is requested. Instead of a nganga in tribal headdress he sees a more prosaic figure, the general practitioner, who asks for a psychiatrist to visit. He, in turn, makes a diagnosis of schizophrenia and recommends admission to hospital. If the young man refuses he is likely to be admitted compulsorily so it is unwise for him to argue. It would be wrong to compare the rights and wrongs of each system of assessment and management of this disorder, but the examples illustrate how much of mental symptomatology depends on cultural background and the accepted norms of society. To take another example, previously, in the USSR society learned to respect the State and this was normally considered above criticism. Those who not only criticized it but did so publicly, were highly unusual people. They knew it was an offence against the State punishable by law and there was no immediate benefit in making the criticism. The authorities responded frequently by replacing law with medicine. Psychiatrists were called to see the dissident (in Western eyes), or deviant (in Eastern ones), as he or she must be abnormal to make such heinous allegations. A suitable diagnosis was found, the most common being 'sluggish schizophrenia', and treatment in a psychiatric hospital, sometimes for several years, was arranged (Bloch & Reddeway 1980).

In the United Kingdom most people criticized the State at some time or another; it is often a sign of political maturity to do so. We therefore shudder in horror at the thought that some people are regarded as mad if they act in the same way in another country. But we should not be too complacent. Society determined what is acceptable and this cannot be exported to a different society. Have you noticed, for example, that attacks on and threats to politicians are treated as acceptable or dealt with according to the normal process of law, whereas similar action taken against members of the Royal family is more likely to lead to incarceration in a psychiatric hospital. Are antiroyalists madder than other protesters? Or is it something to do with the rules of society?

The social model reminds us that all symptoms and behaviour have to be considered in the context of the society from which they emanate. This will not only mould and modify the mental abnormalities but also determine the boundary line between normal and abnormal. We must be careful not to pretend that there is some independent objective criterion of mental disorder that is unaffected by these external factors. Our relationship with other people is heavily dependent on social factors although we would prefer not to admit it to ourselves. The story is often told of the police officer who hails a taxi for a drunk and delinquent upper-class fellow in a smart suit, and yet immediately afterwards calls in reinforcements to deal with a working-class drunk with an incomprehensible regional accent. Doctors can also be affected by this and diagnose the former as 'social drinking' and the latter as 'alcohol dependence'.

TREATMENT

By seeing a psychiatric patient as a temporarily misplaced unit in society the social model avoids the tendency to ascribe illness, adherent in other models. The aim is to help the individual to take up an acceptable role again, not to correct a biochemical disturbance, exorcize an unresolved conflict or recondition behaviour.

This requires sensitivity and understanding. In the case of the young man who has just taken the overdose it may be a great mistake to admit him to hospital for 'further observation'. This will give the medical and nursing staff more time to assess him at their leisure but the very act of admitting him may do more harm than they can ever hope to remedy. It could confirm his view of himself as a failure in life as well as adding an extra dimension, that of being loony and being sent to the 'funny farm'. This could increase his estrangement from his family and friends and magnify his already serious depressive symptoms.

He needs an approach to treatment that will improve his self-image and show that he is not to blame for the troubles that have befallen him. They have happened because our current society is at odds with itself. It continues to extol the work ethic yet is readily removing work from all except the highly skilled, its pace of change has accelerated and many unwitting victims have been left behind. He is not to blame for this. His forced unemployment is responsible and has already been shown to create depression and increase suicidal behaviour (Platt 1984).

Once he, and his girlfriend, realize that happiness does not necessarily depend on work, that he can be occupied and productive whether or not he is employed, and that he can earn respect from others through his attitude and behaviour, not just through his social status, he can leave his depression behind. This can be achieved by single or joint interviews or sometimes in groups with othes having similar problems. Such treatment may be given by professionals in a day hospital or by self-help groups in extra-hospital premises; it does not matter so long as he feels at home and can discuss his problems freely and with understanding.

No special attention is given to past problems or hidden conflicts. Introduction of depth psychologies will only make him uncomfortable and distract attention from his present difficulties. These difficulties are not directly of his own making although they are reinforced by his misinterpretation of them.

In some cases more specialized assistance may be necessary. We have discussed already the importance of social roles. Life is a drama and to succeed you need to have acting skills. Many lack the social skills that are necessary for them to fill the role for which they are chosen. We all have to appear confident and in control at times when we have no idea what we are doing, and to talk freely when we do not feel like saying a word. We also have to appear to people in a way that reflects our competence and abilities. Unfortunately many people, and this particularly includes psychiatric patients, lack these abilities or have let them decay over the years. This is particularly likely to happen after prolonged institutional care. Formal teaching of social skills is an important part of rehabilitating

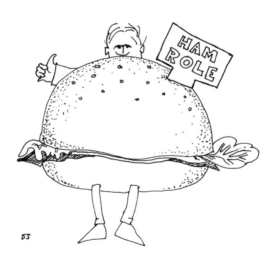

such patients and for helping individuals such as our young man who lacks self-confidence after repeatedly coming off second best in his encounters with the rest of society.

There are twin aims in treatment with the social model. The first is to demonstrate to the patient that many of the fixed views that people hold about their condition are forced on them by society and for which they are not responsible. The second is to allow the patient to develop his or her own opinions and feelings free from the yoke of social pressures. In places like therapeutic communities patients still adopt their own social structure and this is quite often independent of that of society outside. They quickly learn that naked selfishness is not the way to run any form of community and that certain codes of conduct are necessary. However, these are not imposed externally but developed by the patients empirically. Those that work are reinforced and those that lead to conflict are abandoned.

The social model takes a broader view of psychiatric disorder than any other model. To use the analogy of a man looking down a microscope to study an illness; the disease, psychodynamic and behavioural models are all concerned with microscopic details of structure, dynamic change and activity. The patient is being studied closely but in isolation. However, in the social model, not only is the patient being studied under the microscope, but also the doctor. The scope is even larger, because the system whereby objects have to be examined under microscopes is also encompassed in the model.

We mentioned earlier the need for society to have doctors and patients and, accordingly, to set up roles for each of them. First of all, society sets up rules by which some problems are classified as suitable to be dealt with by law and others are regarded as mental illness. Doctors are appointed with interest and expertise in mental health (really mental ill-health). Although, like all doctors, their first duty is to the patient's welfare they also have a duty to society. Although the doctor likes to convince himself that he always thinks of the patient first, in practice society's needs always win.

In 1938 Patrick Hamilton wrote a play called *Gaslight*. The plot concerns the admission of a lady against her will to a mental hospital. She is no longer wanted by her husband and various tricks are played on her in an attempt to make out she is mentally ill. There is a family history of mental disturbance and her husband plays on this, making out to the medical authorities that his wife has also become mentally disturbed. By securing her admission to mental hospital he is free to go off with another woman. Throughout the play we are left in no doubt that the unfortunate victim is continuously sane.

This is not a fanciful idea. The 'Gaslight phenomenon', as it has been named, is now well described in the psychiatric literature (Barton & Whitehead 1969, Smith & Sinanan 1972, Lund & Gardiner 1977), and is now so pervasive that it is no longer worthy of published record. When people deviate from the accepted norms of behaviour they are often labelled 'mad' because this leads to a suitable mode of disposal. No one questions the motives of society; all is subservient to the scrutiny of the patient and his so-called abnormalities. If society, whether in the form in its smallest unit, the family, or its largest, the community, perceives the patient as a nuisance the wheels of control are set in motion and institutional care is arranged. It is very difficult to reverse this process and all doctors working in psychiatric hospitals know many patients who have no significant mental disturbance but stay in hospital because they have nowhere else go.

Psychiatrists are the only doctors with the power to take away people's liberty. This is an exceptional power and society is a little wary of those who possess it. For this reason it is important for the public to think of psychiatrists as rather strange but non-threatening figures, who talk vaguely and largely incomprehensively. It suits society to label most psychiatrists as advocates of the psychodynamic model, as these odd people in search of the *id* seem far removed from the machinery of state. In fact, all psychiatrists are in a sense agents of the State unless they practise privately or in specialties such as psychotherapy where these issues are largely avoided.

The advocate of the social model may feel it necessary to go beyond helping his patients to understand how society influences and perpetuates psychological distress. They may also feel it necessary to try and alter the way society deals with the mentally ill by changing social attitudes. A single-minded social psychiatrist in Italy, Franco Basaglia, did just this. He came to regard psychiatric hospitals as instruments of 'social violence' that led to patients being excluded from normal society. The answer was to close the mental hospitals. After dramatically reducing the inpatient population of the San Giovanni mental hospital in Trieste in northern Italy from 1200 to 350 patients in eight years he started a political movement that became so influential that the government was forced to act. A law was passed in 1978 which forbade the admission of any new patients to mental hospitals and arranged instead for them to be seen at special psychiatric admission units in general hospitals.

Basaglia died in 1982 but his work goes on. Although the reform has been heavily criticized (Jones & Poletti 1985) no adequate data have been provided to support such criticisms. Indeed, in an influential review of the Italian experience, Tansella & Williams (1987)

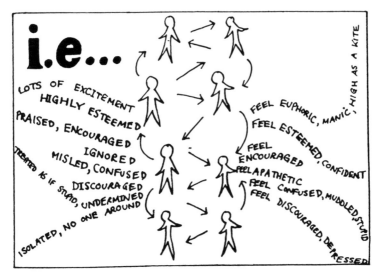

conclude that 'in places where the reform has been properly implemented, the Italian model of community care without mental hospitals is able to cope with the problems presented by the whole range of psychiatric patients resident in a catchment area'. The Italians have reminded us forcefully that all psychiatry has sociopolitical overtones and unless we are fully in tune with the social model we will go astray.

Family therapy (Barker 1981) has been an important development in psychiatry. While developed to a large extent by psychodynamic psychiatrists it was also pioneered by social and anthropological scientists, and is closely related conceptually to these fields. The family approach takes the family as the key social group, and regards the family system as powerfully influential in allotting and maintaining the roles of individual members of it. Some family therapists use a psychodynamic model to understand and interpret feelings generated in the family group, but others are more influenced by a model based on general systems theory (Von Bertalanffy 1968) in which the social dynamics of the family system result in family members taking on various moods, behaviour patterns, and roles, including the sick role.

REFERENCES

Ambelas, A. (1979) Psychologically stressful events in the precipitation of manic episodes. *British Journal of Psychiatry*, **135**, 15–21.

Barker, P. (1981) *Basic Family Therapy*. Granada, London.

Barton, R. and Whitehead, T.A. (1969) The gaslight phenomenon. *Lancet*, **i**, 1258–1260.

Bloch, S. and Reddeway, P. (1980). *Russia's Political Hospitals: Abuse of Psychiatry in the Soviet Union* , Gollancz, London.

Brown, G.W. and Birley, J.L.T. (1968) Crises and life events and the onset of schizophrenia. *Journal of Health and Social Behaviour*, **9**, 203–214.

Brown, G.W. and Harris, T. (1978) *The Social Origins of Depression*. Tavistock Press, London.

Cooper, B. and Sylph, J. (1973) Life events and the onset of neurotic illness: an investigation in general practice. *Psychological Medicine*, **3**, 421–435.

Durkheim, E. (1897) *Le Suicide*. Alcan, Paris.

Finlay-Jones, R. and Brown, G.W. (1981) Types of stressful life events and the onset of anxiety and depressive disorders. *Psychological Medicine*, **11**, 803–815.

Hamilton, P. (1938) *Gaslight*. Constable, London.

Holmes, T.H. and Rahe, R.H. (1967) The social readjustment rating scale. *Journal of Psychosomatic Research*, **11**, 213–218.

Jones, K. and Poletti, A. (1985) Understanding the Italian experience. *British Journal of Psychiatry*, **146**, 341–347.

Lund, C.K. and Gardiner, A.Q. (1977) The gaslight phenomenon—an institutional variant. *British Journal of Psychiatry*, **131**, 533–534.

Parkes, C.M., Benjamin, B. and Fitzgerald, R.G. (1967) Broken heart: a statistical survey of increased mortality among widowers. *British Medical Journal*, **1**, 740–743.

Paykel, E.S., Myers, J.K., Diendelt, M.N., Klerman, G.L., Lindenthal, J.J. and Pepper, M.P. (1969) Life events and depression: a controlled study. *Archives of General Psychiatry*, **21**, 753–760.

Paykel, E.S., Prusoff, B.A. and Uhlenhuth, E.H. (1971) Scaling of life events. *Archives of General Psychiatry*, **25**, 340–347.

Platt, S. (1984) Unemployment and suicidal behaviour: a review of the literature. *Social Science and Medicine*, **19**, 93–115.

Smith, C.G. and Sinanan, K. (1972) The 'gaslight phenomenon' reappears. *British Journal of Psychiatry*, **120**, 685–686.

Szasz, T.S. (1961) *The Myth of Mental Illness*. Harper and Row, New York.

Tansella, M. and Williams, P. (1987) The Italian experience and its implications. *Psychological Medicine*, **17**, 283–289.

Totman, R. (1979) *Social Causes of Illness*. Souvenir Press, London.

Vaughn, C.E. and Leff, J.P. (1973) The influence of family and social factors on the course of psychiatric illness: a comparison of schizophrenic and depressed neurotic outpatients. *British Journal of Psychiatry*, **129**, 125–137.

Von Bertalanffy, L. (1968) *General Systems Theory*. George Brazillier, New York.

FURTHER READING

Bhugra, D. and Leff, J. (eds) (1992) *Principles of Social Psychiatry*. Blackwell, Oxford.

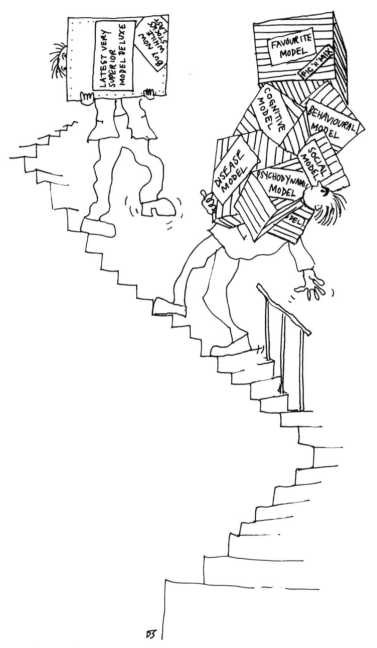

'. . . will fall over backwards to say they are eclectic . . .'

CHAPTER 7

Working Models in Practice

Much of the discussion and argument has been about which of the models described in previous chapters are most appropriate for psychiatry. In general, biologically orientated psychiatrists prefer the disease model, the private psychotherapist prefers the psychodynamic model or variations of it extending through to the cognitive model, psychologists split almost equally between those who follow the behavioural and dynamic models, and the epidemiologist often prefers the social model. If you challenge each of these professionals directly, however, they will fall over backwards to say that they are eclectic, that they use several models at different times and are prepared to use these flexibly to suit the circumstances. We do not deny that they intend to use these models in this way but in practice very few do, and when you find someone who adheres absolutely to one model, such as the well-known psychologist, Hans Eysenck, does the behavioural one, it is only achieved by abstinence from actual clinical contact. When exposed at the coal-face of clinical practice single models just do not work.

A source of confusion in trying to understand psychiatry and construct models of the subject is the notion that there is an underlying psyche, or mind, which can be diagnosed, treated and cured. Of course the concept of mind is useful, but mainly in the healthy sense, and in mental illness its complexities are more to the fore. In Fig. 7.1 the interrelationships between the different levels of function are illustrated. This is just as complex and ambiguous as many world events and is best conceived as an interplay between various organizational levels.

For example, let us consider the problems of a young man with an intellectual handicap due to brain injury at birth. What is 'wrong'

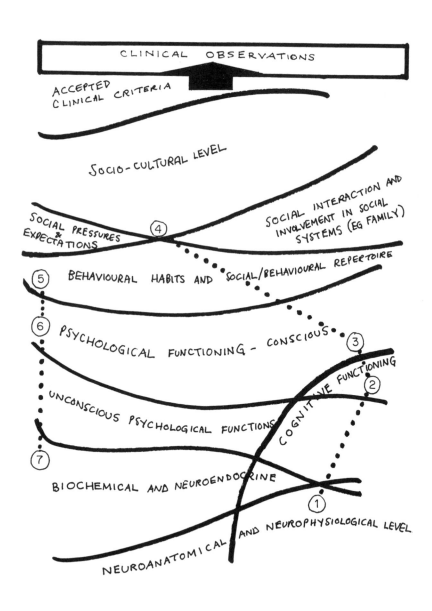

Fig 7.1   Levels of functioning

with him, a necessary description before effective care can be given, could be described in terms of (see 1–4 in Figure 7.1):

1. Damaged neural connections.
2. Problems in learning.
3. Low self-esteem.
4. Conflict between his abilities and those imposed by normal social expectations.

The 'lesion' may be a neurological one but the management involves far more than a knowledge of pathophysiology—training, family attitudes and individual feelings are all part of the strategy of treatment. Similarly, a young woman with a social phobia appears to have a straightforward problem involving social behaviour and psychological perception, but at various times it can be aggravated by biochemical factors affecting her general mood (e.g. premenstrual exacerbation of symptoms and enhancement by coincidental depression) (5, 6 and 7 in Figure 7.1).

Nevertheless, most practitioners feel comfortable with one of the five models we have described and attempt, like Procrustes, to fit their patients' problems to their favourite model wherever possible. It is only when this does not work that they will look elsewhere and, somewhat reluctantly, apply the approaches from other models.

This is particularly evident when there is a multi-disciplinary review of a difficult clinical problem. Each practitioner slants the discussion in favour of his or her preferred model and a power struggle develops between them. The approach chosen is usually that preferred by the dominant figure in the discussion and, to some extent, the others tend to go away dissatisfied. It would be wrong to say that this is a common outcome of attempts at multi-disciplinary working in psychiatry. There is a genuine wish to reach consensus but each member, not always consciously, is fighting the corner of one model against the others.

In fact, to paraphrase the Dodo in Lewis Carroll's *Alice Through the Looking Glass*, 'all models have won and all should have prizes'. All that is needed is to select the appropriate model and the appropriate time. Thus it is acknowledged that every patient needing mental health care is (a) a biological entity with biochemical, pathophysiological, pharmacological and, sometimes, anatomical changes occurring because of their mental state abnormality, (b) that their disorder has important social and environmental associations, (c) that they are emotional beings who have many feelings expressed and unexpressed and which often conflict, and (d) that they have distressing thoughts and behaviour that are maladaptive.

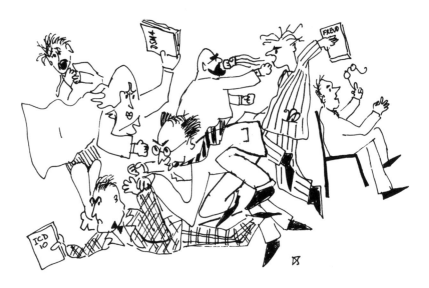

'The approach chosen is usually that preferred by the dominant figure in the discussion . . .'

In deciding which model to use we first of all need to have a common procedure to place an individual's problem at the appropriate model. We then match treatment and other forms of management with that model, often bringing into operation the approaches of other models where necessary. A common procedure is that of diagnosis, a discipline which tends to be confined to medical members of the psychiatric team but is increasingly being recognized as necessary for all mental health practitioners.

DIAGNOSIS IN PSYCHIATRY

In general medicine and surgery one diagnosis usually suffices; indeed some teachers advise never to make more than one. In psychiatry single diagnoses are less common, but we are getting more efficient in making them. It is a mark of the progress made in psychiatry in recent years that many diagnoses have been refined to such an extent that an increasing number of people throughout different countries and cultures can agree on a common language to describe mental disorders. Diagnosis is embodied in two classification systems, the International Classification of Disease

(ICD), which has just undergone its 10th revision (ICD-10), and the Diagnostic and Statistical Manual for mental disorders (DSM), which is close to publishing its fourth revision (DSM-IV). These classifications are published by the World Health Organisation (1992) and the American Psychiatric Association (1987) respectively.

Many psychiatric disorders do not have clean diagnostic descriptions but this does not mean that diagnosis is a waste of time. It is worth while examining one of the classifications, ICD-10, to show its value for each of the models described in the previous chapters. Diagnoses are useful because they allow mental health professionals and research workers to know what each is talking about so that each has a common frame of reference and because they are useful shorthand for groups of disorders which share the same clinical features, and have similar outcomes and agreed treatments. The main diagnoses in ICD-10 are shown in Table 7.1.

A good diagnosis carves nature at its joints so that each condition stands alone in splendid isolation from its fellows. Very few psychiatric diagnoses do this but it does not mean they should be abandoned as useless or regarded merely as labels that only serve to stigmatize patients and minimize the special features of each problem that make it unique. Those who criticize diagnosis and use other systems (of which perhaps the most popular are those based on problem-orientation) will realize that although there are some advantages in their approach, there is considerable economy in transmitting information when it can be simplified to straightforward diagnostic terms.

Sometimes this can only be done by using more than one diagnosis and deciding, somewhat arbitrarily, that one should take precedence over the others. Thus from Table 7.1 it is easy to see how some patients can have diagnoses from several categories. Consider, for example, a young man whom one of us saw recently in hospital after breaking his leg following a fall when he was drunk. (The different diagnoses from ICD-10 are indicated in italics during the description and the detailed coding also given.) He was seen shortly after he had returned from the operating theatre where he had received a general anaesthetic during the treatment of an open fracture in which full cleaning (debridement) of the wound was considered necessary because of the fear of gangrene. After recovering from the anaesthetic he was confused and disorientated and muttered nonsensical replies to questions. *Diagnosis in F0 category—delirium (05.0).* Although it was impossible to get a detailed history about his problem he admitted to heavy alcohol consumption, mainly beer, over the previous six years. Whenever he stopped

Table 7.1   Summary of Chapter 5 of the 10th revision of the International Classification of Diseases

Main category	Sub-categories	Main features
Organic (F0)	Dementias Delirium Mental disorders due to physical disease Personality or behaviour disorder due to brain disease or injury	Conditions in which brain dysfunction is present, and manifested by disturbances of cognition, mood, perception or behaviour
Psychoactive substance use (F1)	States of intoxication, harmful use, dependence and withdrawal states, and psychosis resulting from use of alcohol, opioids, cannabis, sedatives, cocaine, tobacco, halluncinogens and other drugs	Includes all mental disorders which are considered to be a direct consequence of drug use and which would not have occurred without consumption of the drug (or drugs)
Schizophrenia, schizotypal and delusional disorders (F2)	Schizophrenia Schizotypal disorder Persistent delusional disorders Acute and transient psychotic disorders Schizoaffective disorders	Conditions in which there are distortions of thinking, perception and mood not due to an organic condition and which are most prominent in schizophrenia
Mood (affective) disorders (F3)	Manic episodes Depressive episodes Bipolar affective disorder Recurrent depressive disorder Persistent affective disorders	A range of disorders in which disturbance of mood (affect) is the main feature, together with other symptoms which are easily understood in the context of change of mood and activity
Neurotic, stress-related and somatoform disorders (F4)	Phobic disorder Other anxiety disorders Obsessive-compulsive disorder Stress and adjustment disorders Dissociative and conversion disorders Somatoform disorders	A group of disorders in which certain symptoms, historically recognized as part of 'neurosis', are most marked and which may have a psychological causation

Table 7.1 *cont.*

Main category	Sub-categories	Main features
Behavioural syndromes and mental disorders associated with physio- logical dys- function and hormone imbalance (F5)	Eating disorders Psychogenic sleep disorders Sexual dysfunctions Mental disorders associated with the puerperium	Disorders in which physiological and hormonal factors may be involved in causation or be prominent in association with the disorder
Disorders of adult personality and behaviour (F6)	Personality disorder Enduring personality change Habit and impulse disorders Gender identity disorders Sexual preference disorders	Conditions of clinical significance in which behaviour patters tend to be persistent and which are 'the expression of the individual's characteristic life-style and mode of relating to self and others'
Mental retardation (F7)	Mild mental retardation Moderate mental retardation Severe mental retardation Profound mental retardation Other types of mental retardation	A condition of 'arrested or incomplete development of the mind', manifest by impairment of skills commonly associated with intelligence
Disorders of psychological development (F8)	Developmental disorders of speech and language Specific developmental disorder of scholastic skills Specific developmental dis- order of motor function Pervasive developmental disorders (e.g. autism)	Conditions that begin in infancy or childhood, delay in the development of functions related to maturation of the nervous system, and which generally have a steady rather than remitting course
Behavioural and emotional disorders with onset occurring in childhood or adolescence (F9)	Hyperkinetic disorder Conduct disorder Mixed disorder of conduct and emotions Emotional disorder of childhood Disorders of social function (childhood) Tic disorders Other behavioural or emotional disorders	A mixture of disorders in which the only common features are an onset early in life and a fluctuating or unpredictable course

Taken from Chapter 5 of the 10th revision of the International Classification of Diseases (ICD-10) (Reproduced by permission of the World Health Organisation 1992) drinking for more than 12 hours he developed severe stomach pains and a craving for alcohol. *Diagnosis in F1 category—alcohol dependence syndrome (10.2)*. On questioning him about his reason for heavy alcohol consumption he admitted to persistent, relatively mild depression which he claimed was dulled to some extent by drinking and therefore made bearable. However, even when drunk, he still felt depressed to some extent. *Diagnosis F3— dysthymic disorder (34.1)*. He also complained that he was anxious for much of the time because he had no confidence in his dealings with other people and felt that people were scrutinizing him closely whenever he met with them. He felt very embarrassed among groups of people that he did not know and tried to avoid such groups wherever possible. *Diagnosis F4—social phobia (40.1)*. On enquiring about his background it was clear that he had been unsettled in his personal relationships ever since adolescence. He was excessively dependent on his mother and, despite several attempts to leave home he always returned to her care. He relied excessively on her although he had confidence to go out and meet other people when he had a few drinks. *Diagnosis F6—dependent personality disorder (60.7)*. During his childhood he had been a slow developer and had been protected by his parents to a greater extent than the other two children in the family, partly because he was more anxious than the other children. He also wet his bed at night on average 5–10 times each month until the age of 12. This had been investigated in hospital without any organic cause being found. *Diagnosis F9—non-organic enuresis (98.0)*.

Each of these diagnoses has a clear description associated with diagnostic guidelines. When they have been diagnosed correctly a great deal more information is conveyed to the listener or reader who knows the detailed criteria for the diagnoses. Although it is possible to make fun of the list of diagnoses in the patient described above, if we opted for economy and listed all these diagnoses it would convey at least as much information as the long prose account above and would be much easier to collect and code. Diagnosis in psychiatry, like diagnosis in any branch of medicine, is simply a form of shorthand between informed people, and like most shorthand, it does not look pretty but is effective for communication.

Let us look at the process of diagnosis in practice. The assessment usually proceeds in three steps, two *descriptive* and the third *explanatory*. The explanatory step is not a statement of observable facts but a working hypothesis about the nature of the disorder, and this is the step where the various models for mental disorder are invoked.

Step 1

This is a simple account of the reason for referral and in literal terms is the proper use of problem-orientation (e.g. 'I can't sleep, I don't get on with people, I get no enjoyment out of life, people are persecuting me'). Sometimes the reasons for referral are much more complex, and include many more people, and in such cases it may be appropriate to ask the question 'Who is complaining about what?' (Steinberg 1983).

Step 2

This is to identify an accepted clinical psychiatric disorder, if there is one. *Not all problems presented to the psychiatrist necessarily include an individual with a psychiatric disorder.* It is not always helpful to label an unhappy or worried or misbehaving person 'depressed', 'anxious' or 'sociopathic' for example, unless their feelings or misbehaviour really amount to psychiatric disorder. However, this is a very large topic that cannot be taken further here. Those who would like to pursue this ethical–philosophical point should read further (Foucault 1967, Szasz 1961, Lewis 1953, and Ramon 1985, among others).

Step 3

This is the construction of a working hypothesis about the nature of the problem. It is at this stage that we attempt, relying more on clinical experience than hard evidence, to give due weight to the various possible components of a patient's case. One person's distress may seem to be caused and maintained by present circumstances; another by the impact in the present of past experiences; another by the influence of their physiological state and genetic inheritance. On this basis we would have to make decisions about the sort of approach most likely to help: social help, behavioural training, individual psychotherapy, family therapy or medication.

Two characteristics of psychiatric assessment need to be mentioned at this point. The first is the increase in tendency for classification to use multi-axial approaches in which clinical diagnosis is only one part. In the American Classification of Mental Disorders (DSM-II-R) the clinical diagnosis is axis 1, personality status is described in axis 2, and developmental delay, intellectual status, physical health, social functioning and reactions to stress are all separate axes. This allows the use of several different 'labels' which do not contradict each other. The second characteristic is the use of a *diagnostic formulation*, a statement that incorporates all the three steps described above and also incorporates a multi-axial approach in those cases.

Step 1

A man is referred by the Casualty Department after an overdose. He has no general practitioner. He lives along but was taken to hospital by his landlord who thinks 'something should be done' and is anxious that there is no recurrence. His only relatives are in Scotland, and do not know about what happened.

Step 2

On examination he has depressed mood, is actively thinking about suicide, and has additional symptoms of disturbed sleep, loss of interest, appetite and weight loss, and hopelessness about the future that lead to a diagnosis of depressive illness.

Step 3

This man has become depressed this time because of the loss of his job. He is significantly depressed at present and may require anti-depressant drugs. At the same time, however, his capacity to use counselling or psychotherapy should be explored because it is likely that his emotional experiences in childhood have made him extremely vulnerable to major changes and losses in life. Whatever the usefulness of medication or psychotherapy, his social isolation and poor social skills mean that his unemployment may well become chronic, and occupational and social assessment and help will both be needed. While these are being explored, he will need close observation because his mental state, social isolation and history make him a high risk for a further suicidal attempt. The feasibility and usefulness of discussion things with his landlord, and contacting his relatives, should be explored, with appropriate permissions; and he ought to be registered with a general practitioner.

HOW CAN DIFFERENT MODELS INTERACT?

There is no reason why the quite different conceptual models we have outlined should not interact with each other, and it will be seen that the general approach we are recommending includes looking for such interactions.

Thus there is a well-recognized association between blood lead levels in children and their having educational and behavioural problems; sufficient evidence, it may be said, to justify urgent measures to reduce this atmospheric pollution. However, there is *also* an association between educational and behavioural problems, and living in poor neighbourhoods with poor schooling in inner cities with high local levels of atmospheric lead: e.g. in the shadow of motorways. Here we see socio-economic (and indeed political) factors interacting with children's behavioural and educational performance and their neurophysiological status.

Yet another example is the simple behavioural model by which a patient develops a phobia for a situation in which he or she had a bad experience: perhaps a fear of flying conditioned by a near-accident. In clinical practice such clear-cut causes are unusual. What is more often seen is the development of anxiety (or other persisting distress) in a situation which *for that individual* was unusually highly disturbing. Thousands of people may have the same experience (e.g. discomfort in crowds) without developing symptoms that persist and become disabling. A few, however, develop a phobic state. Is this because some people become more highly aroused than others in crowded circumstances? Is this because some are physiologically different, (i.e. more vulnerable to maladaptive learning)? Or is it because for some their emotional development gives a highly anxiety-laden *personal meaning* to the situation? Since not everyone responds in the same way, there is clearly a personal characteristic or set of characteristics interposed between stimulus and response. In some people this may be their physiological learning set, in others it may be unconscious determinants of what they find particularly frightening, and in others it may be determined by personality status. We see no problem in hypothesizing that both psychodynamic and physiological factors can influence the individual response to a situation, although the degree to which each operates in the individual case will vary.

THE MEDICAL MODEL

The reader may wonder how we have come so far without describing the best-known (and much maligned) model of all. We believe

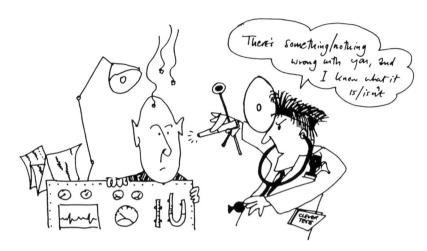

'The Medical Model'

the term 'medical model' is widely misused and misunderstood, and in particular that it is erroneous to equate it with the disease model. As we mentioned in the introduction, we have not used this description because of confusion surrounding the adjective 'medical'. The pedigree of the 'medical model' is not to be found in the annals of discovery about the physical origins and treatment of disease, but in the nature of the doctor–patient relationship. This relationship has archetypal qualities quite distinct from other professional relationships. In it (a) the physician, purports to diagnose disorder or its absence in (b) the patient, by using an understanding of symptoms and signs and their implications.

Other professional–client relationships are quite different. The craftsman does something for other people, whether it is putting up a shelf or designing a bathroom. The lawyer acts as the client's advocate, putting his or her case in the best possible way, whatever its merits or demerits. The policeman stops people doing things that the Law says they should not do. We would argue that a psychotherapist or social worker who identifies neurotic conflict 'in' a client and proceeds to treat this 'anomaly' is using the medical model. On the other hand a family therapist or social worker who believes that the problem is not in the individual but in the family group is taking a genuinely different approach.

The medical model, by our definition, is one in which the *diagnosis of individual disorder* is central, whatever the conceptual model of individual disorder is used: disease model, psychodynamic model, cognitive model, behavioural model or some of the social models. It is a pragmatic rather than an ideologically pure model, and, annoying though this may be for purists, quite ready to ditch models of assessment and management if they do not work, and adopt or adapt methods that do. Even worse for the orthodoxies, it is prepared to use one model for diagnosis and another for treatment: thus we may believe that the nature of a patient's anxiety is best understood in psychodynamic terms, but behaviour therapy is the most effective treatment. Or, that the nature of a retarded child's major incapacity is neurophysiological, but the treatment of a mixture of education, social skills training and family work—which may well include working psychodynamically with the parents' distress and disappointment.

In the following pages we describe how each of the five models described earlier in this book can be used effectively and in harmony with other models.

MATCHING MODELS TO DISORDER

How can we combine these models so that they co-exist peacefully? At first sight this may seem difficult. How can symptoms be thought of as disorders in their own right (behavioural model), consequences of irrational thinking (cognitive model), the products of social forces (social model), smoke screens that obscure the true psychic conflict (psychodynamic model), and the building blocks of illness syndromes (disease model) all at the same time? It is true that this cannot be done for the whole range of mental disorder and distress, but you will have noticed already that each model illuminates a corner of psychiatry better than others. The disease model is particularly appropriate for the psychoses (i.e. manic depressive illness, schizophrenia and the organic illnesses with psychiatric symptoms) in which identifiable disease already exists.

The psychodynamic model helps to understand aspects of both normal behaviour and symptomatology that otherwise appear meaningless. The social model shows that mentally ill people, particularly those with neurosis and personality disorders, cannot be considered in isolation from their families, social and cultural background. The behavioural model is at its best in explaining and treating some aspects of neurotic illness that lead to abnormal patterns of behaviour, and the cognitive model shows the importance of irrational thoughts in much of mental illness.

At another level, the behavioural and disease models are particularly orientated towards focused treatment, and the social and psychodynamic models towards understanding the cause of mental illness, although they also incorporate therapy. The different treatments in psychiatry align themselves nicely alongside the models. Physical treatment such as drug therapy, electroconvulsive therapy (ECT) and psychosurgical operations are involved with the disease model; psychotherapy with the psychodynamic model; rehabilitation, social skills training and social engineering (which is part of sociology, economics and politics) with the social model; cognitive therapy with the cognitive model; and behaviour therapy based on learning theory with the behavioural model. If the divisions were mutually exclusive there would be less conflict between the different models but because they overlap argument begins; the psychotherapist believes the behaviourist and the 'organic' psychiatrist are missing aspects of their patients' cases; and vice versa. This is a clinical and ideological concern. When it comes to how much each model should have on the training curriculum there can be major arguments. For theoretical and academic purposes, it is no bad thing that each model should have its adherents, explorers and teachers. For good clinical practice, research purposes and teaching it is important that the positive features of all the models be taken seriously, because any or all may be helpful for the next patient, whoever is the therapist.

DEGREES OF DISTRESS AND DISORDER

It is worth remembering that mental disorder often develops (or improves) gradually, and at different times the features of illness change. The acutely ill schizophrenic patient with delusions that his mind is being controlled by an alien force may present quite a different picture five years later when he has no florid symptoms but is prevented by apathy, social withdrawal and accommodation problems from returning to the society from which he came. It is useful to consider the different levels of illness and the extent to which they interfere with normal mental function and behaviour, before we look at the application of the models. Even when a disorder does not develop chronologically in this way, some or all of what follows illustrates facets of function and malfunction in mental disorder. The levels extend from mild distress at one end, through to symptoms of behaviour change, and end with disintegration of normal function at the other extreme.

1.   Distress

The person is aware of new mental feelings, often unpleasant, such as sadness, nervousness, tension, puzzlement, irritability and anger.

These are noticed more frequently than normal, and the immediate cause is usually recognizable. For example, what is often called 'postnatal blues' comes into this category. After childbirth there are significant hormonal and other biological changes but these are eclipsed by the radical change of a demanding, vulnerable and time-consuming infant. The mother get short of sleep from frequently nightly interruptions for feeding, stresses develop between mother and father until they adjust to the new arrival, and there are increased domestic demands at a time when quiet recuperation would be more appropriate. The mental distress usually is summed up in the ubiquitous term 'nerves' and is accepted as a transitory phenomenon. These feelings amount to emotional distress but are almost universal, and this distinguishes them from mental disorder. Similarly, the tension and stress of front-line soldiers fighting in two world wars (for example in the Great War, where the attrition of trench warfare seemed bound to produce extremes of mental distress) can be regarded as universal phenomena. In such situations it is abnormal *not* to feel distressed and threatened. The symptoms experienced are usually diffuse and variable and will always improve when the stressor has been removed (if they do not we see the beginnings of mental disorder as opposed to distress).

It is less straightforward when the stressor is an internal one. For example, the mental stresses in the early stages of schizophrenia are of a quite different nature. The sufferer is aware that something odd is going on, a stage sometimes described as 'delusional mood', but cannot be sure of the source of his feelings. He usually finds the answer in the external world in the form of a delusion. However, in the early stages of the condition his emotions are little different from thsoe who are distressed because of external stresses.

2. Symptoms

In this phase the continuing emotional conflict becomes more focused on mental and physical complaints. These sometimes become highly specific and are not so directly associated with a precipitating factor. The sufferer remains aware that his feelings or behaviour differ from normal. In conventional terminology 'insight is maintained' and the person may present quite normally to the world at large because he aspires towards normal functioning and tries to compensate for his disability. At this stage, too, the symptoms do not affect behaviour significantly so general observation reveals nothing amiss. Most so-called neurotic symptoms come into this stage; the fears of the agoraphobic, the constant preoccupations of the ruminating obsessional, the despair of the depressed, the preoccupations of the hypochondriac and the panic attacks of anxiety states are all symptomatically equivalent. Unlike the symptoms in the first stage these feelings are not explicable as universal reactions; they are shown only by a minority and occur inappropriately. Apart from these specific symptoms the sufferer functions fairly well and high mental organization is retained except for short periods during the worst symptoms. People at this stage rarely find it helps to remove an apparently precipitating cause. They carry their troubles with them; a simple change of scene, occupation or social contact will not solve the problem.

3.   Irrational Thinking

Once symptoms persist there is the danger that they now become reinforced by distorted thinking. As we noted in Chapter 5, depressed people who withdraw from society can easily develop the 'mental set' that no-one wants to know them, and unexplained panic attacks can be misinterpreted as symptoms of physical disease. This mode of thinking only reinforces the symptoms and so there is a danger they will persist.

4.   Changed Behaviour—Disability and Problems in Relationships

When the symptoms of the third stage become more severe or prolonged there are changes in behaviour. The agoraphobic finds that avoidance of open spaces, supermarkets and public transport is preferable to the fear that these situations arouse. Similarly, the obsessional finds that prolonged and repeated rituals such as hand washing briefly relieve the tension of his constant doubts and ruminations, and the depressed person becomes socially withdrawn and refuses to meet anyone, thereby increasing his isolation and despair. The change in behaviour signals to the outside world that all is not well; a composed exterior does not then disguise the change in behaviour and social functioning. If this change is dramatic enough it can seem to replace the symptoms altogether. For example, agoraphobia, which is more common in women, can develop to the point of complete avoidance of the outside world. In this grossly socially handicapped state, the person concerned may be symptom-free.

Now someone cannot change to this degree without other people being involved too. To remain (as in this case) housebound, other members of the patient's circle, usually his or her family, make adjustments too. The decision of, say, the husband of an agora-phobic woman to 'put up with it', organize himself and the children to do the shopping, is an adjustment, and it may be reasonably asked whether this response is helpful or not.

Other forms of abnormal behaviour are also included in this stage whether or not they are associated with symptoms. This varies from such basic problems as difficulty in self-feeding by mentally handi-capped children to more complex actions such as persistent truant-ing or repeated acts of self-injury. The behaviour is considered to be abnormal because it is counterproductive or even damaging—it does not solve the problem in any way and may even make it worse. You will notice that this stage differs from the earlier ones in that the patient is not necessarily seeking help because of unpleasant feel-ings. Abnormal behaviour may not be regarded as abnormal by the person showing it, and other people—'society'—may be the chief instigators in trying to alter the behaviour. This introduces an ethical aspect of management which does not necessarily apply in the ear-lier stages.

Thus we see that when behaviour is out of the ordinary, for what-ever reason, social functioning and relationships, from the closest family matters to more remote cultural and social expectations, are drawn in.

5.   Disintegration

In the earlier stages the person is capable of a wide range of normal function outside a specific area of malfunction or handicap. At the fifth level of mental disorder this boundary is reduced or even re-moved. The abnormality is so major that it can affect all mental activity. Thinking, feelings and behaviour are all affected and the personality appears to undergo dramatic changes. The imprecise term, psychosis, is usually used for disorders of this degree. As mental function becomes globally disordered, personal awareness of illness is often lost as well. Because of this absence of insight, treatment without the patient's permission is sometimes needed, introducing ethical issues. Because the person's view of the world is no longer determined by reality, he develops false beliefs (delu-sions), incorrect perceptions (illusions and hallucinations), and may feel he no longer has any control over his own mental function, which seems to have passed to an outside agency (passivity feelings and delusions of control). Such features may develop in part from the person's attempt to rationalize the irrational. If the world does not make sense there has to be an internal restructuring to give it some sort of order, although this tends to become one which other people cannot share. In the face of such disorganization all semblance of integrated function disappears. Normal contact through speech and non-verbal communication becomes impossible, important drives such as hunger, thirst and sex become deranged; and hospital admission is often necessary as much to safeguard general health and protect other people as to treat the disorder. When patients with this degree of disorder recover and their view of reality returns to normal they are often unable to remember how they felt when they were ill. This is not surprising, as to reconcile the different perspectives of major illness and good health would require remarkable ingenuity. Perhaps this illustrates best the important qualitative difference between this degree of disorder and the other three; here the psychological experiences are in a different dimension from those of normal experience, neurotic symptoms, cognitive errors and behavioural change.

STAGES IN THE DEVELOPMENT OF MENTAL DISORDER

Obviously there is overlap between the levels of disorder described above, and they cannot be regarded as rigid categories. They are not at the same level as formal diagnoses, and during the course of a single illness any combination of the five may be seen. Let us take, for example, the course of severe depression in a married woman following the death of her husband. Immediately following the loss she goes through a mourning process which is often ritualized, the ritual depending on her cultural background. This may last a few days to several weeks or months. In the first stage the immediate cause of the depressive symptoms is obvious, and if normal grieving can take place amidst a caring group of friends and relatives a healthy adjustment can be made to the loss. If normal grieving is arrested or inhibited, she moves into the second, symptomatic stage, when feelings of depression continue to gnaw inwardly, even though by the mechanisms of repression and denial she appears to have adjusted well to the loss and may be complimented on how well she has coped. Indeed a balance between confronting and repressing feelings may be part of healthy adjustment to loss. If she develops a cycle of negative automatic thinking, believing she is partly to blame for her husband's death or that she is just a burden on others, she enters the third stage. Later still, social withdrawal and avoidance herald the hiatrists would see this patient at the fifth level, when her symptoms are established and admisson to hospital is essary because of the danger of successful suicide. It does e a great deal of skill and intellect to appreciate that the e illness is in some way due the bereavement, but at this underlying cause is not of immediate concern. The doctor ith a woman who is a suicidal risk, and possibly at risk of ll health because of poor nutrition and inadequate self- patient is firmly placed in the sick role because she is sick. al function is unbalanced because of the severity of this decisions about treatment will have to be made indepen- not necessarily with the patient's co-operation. Admis- spital and treatment with ECT and antidepressant drugs fore have to be given without her permission. During this ase of treatment the hospital setting and attitudes of other medical and nursing staff are largely immaterial, although become very important as recovery progresses and should ored now.

el—*cognitive model* As the patient's psychotic symptoms the negative thinking behind the depression will become inent. Feelings of guilt, blaming herself for her husband's believing that she cannot live without him, are inap- assumptions that will prolong the depression. The depres- be prevented from returning to its former cognitive 'set' all possibility of improvement is excluded and morbid preoccupies her brain. At a fairly simple level, and cer- which has not required the skills of a cognitive therapist, e ward can explore the patient's feelings and beliefs in a that helps her to understand that she can adjust to the er husband without being a traitor to his memory.

l—*behavioural model* As the patient responds to treat- will lose her delusions and hallucinations but remain so- drawn. She will probably be reluctant to eat regularly and end most of her time alone. During this time there is a at ruminating about her husband will again lead to a evere depressive symptoms. The nursing staff react to this l with a form of operant conditioning. They will posi- force socially outgoing behaviour but will be careful not ely reinforce the withdrawal by any form of punishment ow that this can only reinforce the depression. They will her to eat with other patients, talk to her socially instead formally discussing her symptoms, and praise her when

emergence of the fourth stage. Attempts to adjust to the loss appear to cease altogether and other people are unable to alter her move towards isolation. Finally she develops a depressive psychosis, with delusions of poverty, unworthiness and guilt, accompanied by paranoid ideas and auditory hallucinations of an unpleasant critical kind. These tell her she is useless and that suuicide is the only way out of the burden she is causing to her friends and relatives. At this stage she no longer feels ill but wicked. The characteristic bodily changes of severe depression, including marked loss of weight and appetite, constipation, sleep disturbance with waking in the early hours, and a worsening of her depressed mood with feelings of complete hopelessness and worthlessness are present. As she feels such a burden on everyone and with such low self-esteem it is not surprising that she now contemplates suicide. Meanwhile, she elicits a range of reactions from other people: sympathy, anxiety, sadness, anger and mixed feelings too.

Other disorders may only show obvious evidence of one of these phases, others two or three, but in all instances there is the possibility that the disorder can present at any of the five levels. How can this be explained?

Hierarchy of Models

We are all aware of hierarchies in our lives. We all have to deal with much larger amounts of information than our brains can cope with and we order these in a way that leads to greatest efficiency. In addition to our own internal hierarchies we have external ones, most obvious in the structures of large organizations. Typically the bottom level of the organization contains the most people and the top level the least. A general feature of a hierarchy is that those on higher levels incorporate the characteristics of the lower levels. Thus the chairman of a large international company is regarded as representing the company at all levels. Thus, for example, if there is a major scandal involving a functioning of the lowest level of the organization the chairman may be regarded as responsible and forced to resign even though he had no direct knowledge of the circumstances and personnel involved in the scandal.

Models in psychiatry have a similar hierarchical structure and this is shown in Figure 7.2. The most minor mental illness (e.g. feeling angry and upset after failing a job interview) does not qualify for any diagnostic label but certainly creates social dysfunction and involves the social model. However, when specific symptoms are established at the second level of the hierarchy the psychodynamic

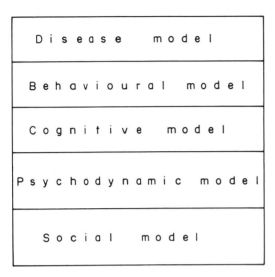

Fig 7.2   A hierarchy of models. Note that this is a true hierarchy in which each higher level comprises its own level and the features of all lower levels

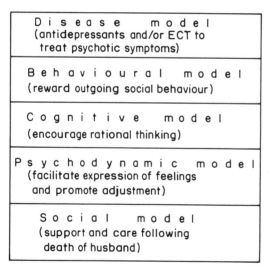

Fig 7.3   Matching models with treatment in Mrs X

model may be used. When maladapti
cognitive model is most appropriate a
mainly in behaviour, the behavioural
leads directly to an appropriate progra
incorporate treatment from the same
with treatment beneath it (Figure 7.3).

Matching Levels and Models

It will not have escaped attention that th
discussed in earlier chapters match the
respects. The hierarchical model states t
atric disorder there is an aprropriate n
that model is only correct for that level
der moves to a different level, another n
used. The level of disorder corresponds
model could be identified as the medic
medical is a comprehensive term used
caring. As pointed out, this term has
quarters as the disease model and for
description as the hierarchical model.

At the first level of illness, which only
of the level of feelings, formal psychiatric
and the social model is appropriate. Wl
established in the second level the pscl
used. When maladaptive behaviour-res
third level, the behavioural model app
thinking is dominant in the fourth level th
The disease model should be reserved for
of the fifth level. Because the different l
different times in the course of an illness
sume that any one model is suitable for a
ertheless, because some disorders predor
one level there will be a tendency for one

In our introduction we emphasized that
they fit the facts closely and provide a cohe
They are practical instruments rather than t
test whether this particular combination of
need to see whether our new correlative
good psychiatric practice and whether it ha

Fifth level—disease model To return to ou
our model help us to understand and treat

Most ps
psychot
often ne
not requ
depress
stage th
is faced
physica
care. Th
Her me
stage a
dently
sion to
may th
disease
patien
they w
not be

Fourth
impro
more
death
propr
sion
in w
think
tainly
staff
gentl
death

Thir
men
ciall
wish
dan
retu
with
tive
to r
as t
enc
of

she achieves small advances such as baking cakes for other patients in the occupational therapy department or takes part in group activities on the ward.

Second level—psychodynamic model As she improves in confidence and can face society again she will move towards the second level. This is the time to explore her thoughts and feelings about her dead husband, knowing that at first this may be a painful process. By 'working through' her loss again she can undergo the normal grieving process and restructure her world in a satisfactory and healthy way. It is likely that this stage could be carried out at a day hospital or in an outpatient clinic after discharge from in-patient care.

First level—social model The first level of disorder would predominate sometime later when she is probably attending as an outpatient to monitor progress. Although she has adjusted in many ways to the loss of her husband she cannot help being reminded of him as she sits in the house where they have spent so many years together. Provided that the treatment at the other four levels has been completed satisfactorily a change of accommodation, preferably to one where she has greater social contacts, is all that is necessary to complete the adjustment and treatment of her depressive illness.

When changing from one approach to another during the course of a disorder one is merely moving to a different level in the hierarchy (Figure 7.3). This is hardly a revolutionary concept but is rarely formalized. In general medicine a condition such as hypertension can be viewed similarly. At level five the important aspect is to bring the blood pressure down by drug therapy or similar medical means, but once this has been achieved the patient needs to have his individual needs and personality considered, and advice given about his lifestyle, occupational pressures and personal relationships, much of which may need to come from non-medical sources.

The hierarchical approach should also predict successfully that when the level of the disorder does not correspond then the approach will be unsuccessful. There is a popular, but now outmoded, view of schizophrenia that it is not a true illness but a natural reaction of man to the oppressive conformity of our society. The victim can only break out of the mould cast for him by society by apparently becoming mad in the form of schizophrenia. This serves as a vehicle to 'break through to health' and therefore, according to the hypothesis, it is best to treat the condition at the first stage of our model by altering society rather than the patient. When this theory has been put to the test the evidence is universally negative. Patients do not achieve health by passing through a schizophrenic illness. If the condition is not treated using the disease model it is likely to become persistent, chronic and damage the personality irreparably. There is similar negative evidence that disorders in the first stage of illness can be treated by the disease stage of our model. It is of no value to treat people distressed and disadvantaged by poverty and poor housing by hospital admission and drug treatment. These changes will temporarily remove the unpleasant feelings but will not alter the underlying difficulties, and by 'medicalizing' the problem the patient may be prevented from taking action himself to change matters.

The demarcation lines are not so clearly drawn when intermediate phases are considered. For example, a severely agoraphobic patient who generally avoids all situations outside the home may be treated according to level three along behavioural lines. Gradual exposure to the feared situation or prevention of conditioned avoidance by remaining in the feared situation until anxiety is resolved may be successful but sometimes fails because of continued anxiety and panic. In the worst form of the disorder the patient has a 'panphobia' of everything and can be said to reach the fifth stage of the model. It is therefore appropriate to give drug treatment to reduce or suppress the panic feelings that are interfering with behaviour therapy. Similarly, a phobic patient who is responding to behaviour therapy may need cognitive therapy to prevent him from developing any new symptoms of anxiety by further phobic avoidance, and he may also need psychotherapeutic intervention to illustrate how the disorder has been manipulated (not necessarily consciously) by either the patient or close relatives for a variety of reasons. Unless this is resolved the phobias may return.

Cause and Pathology

It is possible to match the causes of mental disorder with levels in a similar way to that for treatment, but care is needed in defining cause, or to use its more technical synonym, aetiology. Just as an illness can manifest features of all five levels at different times so can its cause affect all five levels. A distinction is often made between 'causes' and 'triggering events' but this defines the level rather than a fundamental difference. Triggering events are usually at level one in the hierarchical model but they can lead to changes at other levels, and the nature of the disorder is the resultant of all these changes.

It is wrong to define any mental disorder by its apparent cause because of variability in response. Thus the term 'reactive depression' should be discarded because it implies a different type of depression than, for example, so-called 'endogenous depression'. If the 'reaction', whatever its nature, leads to significant deficiency in brain levels of certain amines (5-hydroxy-tryptamine and noradrenaline), then the clinical presentation will be the same as that for the (apparently) endogenously-depressed patient. The reaction has taken place at level one but led to changes at level five, and these determine the nature of the depression.

Most mental disorders are reactive in one sense, in that their timing is determined by one or more external precipitants.

Underlying predisposition, however, really decides the nature of the disorder and it is this level of aetiology that correlates with presentation of illness. Let us take an example to illustrate the importance of underlying predisposition in determining mental illness and how it is linked to aetiology.

Five people, who we shall call A, B, C, D and E, are involved in a road traffic accident but not seriously injured. Subject A is of stable personality and has never had any mental illness. She recovers rapidly from the experience but for a short period prefers to travel by train rather than by car when she has a choice. Subject B is a somewhat insecure anxiety-prone man who has never adjusted to leaving his mother six years previously. He becomes much more anxious after the accident and has acute episodes of panic for no apparent reason. Subject C has a mother who has suffered from agoraphobia when she was a child. She has never had agoraphobia before but after the accident she developed some phobia of car travel. This later generalizes to all travelling outside the house so that she becomes severely agoraphobic. Subject D becomes depressed after the accident and cannot stop ruminating about death and his own mortality. Subject E has a father and grandfather who have had episodes of severe depression and he too has previously been in hospital with episodes of depression and hypomania. He appears not to react to the accident at first but a few weeks later he suddenly becomes overactive and restless, needing little sleep, shows elation and irritability alternately, and plans to build a space ship to take him to Mars as the prospect of continued life on Earth is not exciting.

All these five people have been through the same experience but react differently because of different combinations of aetiological factors. Subject A reacts only to the accident, which can be said to be as much related to social forces as vehicular ones (level one). Subject B reactivates unresolved anxiety that stems from his relationship with his mother (level two). Subject C becomes agoraphobic which generalized avoidance, a pattern of behaviour she has developed at least as much from modelling herself on her agoraphobic mother as a child as on genetic predisposition (level three). Subject D develops persistent depressive thinking. Subject E enters a manic phase (level five) of his manic-depressive illness for which the accident may be seen as an important, though non-specific triggering event. But of course all five (level four) individuals have been through the same experience and so the aetiological factors of the first level are relevant to a varying degree in their resulting problems. Allowing room for simultaneous aetiological factors from different levels removes much of othe controversy about the correct way to regard psychiatric illness. Although a condition may be triggered by social factors that is no reason to regard social forms of management as the only appropriate ones; it is the end result to the triggering that determines the best line of treatment.

Both types of pathology are similarly explained by using the hierarchy. Pathology not only means gross changes in bodily organs such as the loss of brain cells and flattening of the grooves (sulci) in the brain in conditions such as senile dementia; it describes abnormalities at other levels also. So in psychoses well-known phrases such as 'ideas of reference' and 'delusional perception' are examples of descriptive psychopathology, and the maladaptive behaviour patterns of stage three, the dynamic psychopathology of stage two, and the social pathology of stage one are all manifestations of the form of illness. As long as one level of pathology is not applied to an inappropriate stage—for example it would be nonsense to describe someone in a depressive stupor as displaying introjection and repression—then there is no difficulty in fitting pathology to the model.

Prevention

Prevention also follows the multimodel pattern of aetiology. It is appropriate for any preventive measure to be given provided that it matches the mental disorder at one level at least. Thus patients with recurrent episodes of mania and depression may take the treatment from stage five of our model, the drug lithium carbonate, even when they are completely well and outside the scope of our model altogether. But it would be inappropriate to give antidepressant tablets to a population living in squalid stressful conditions on the grounds that it would prevent them from becoming depressed.

How do we go about using the hierarchical approach in practice? First of all there are some parts of each of the models described previously that can be incorporated into our model as general rules. The two aspects of the disease model that apply to all levels of illness are the need for a formalized assessment of every mental problem and the acceptance that in a doctor–patient relationship the patient has to adopt a sick role at some stage, even if it is only at the beginning. The need for a formalized assessment will already be obvious to the reader. This assessment would be usually made at a first interview and involves a judicious mix of direct questions from the interviewer and spontaneous description of problems by the patient. A proper history of the problem and an assessment of the current mental state of the patient are essential parts, for without them much relevant material will remain undetected. The interviewer's assessment will be summarized in a formulation of the problem in aetiological, diagnostic and prognostic terms.

We should also like the doctor to describe which stage of the illness the patient has reached as this will influence management, but as he will look in vain for any indication of this in psychiatric text books we shall have to ask him to use his own judgement in deciding this question. This judgement will require both an objective assessment of the patient's state and a recording of the patient's own views about his attitudes and feelings towards his problem. Sometimes these will vary; the patient may think his attacks of sweating and palpitations signify organic disease whereas the doctor will view them as anxiety symptoms. A sound knowledge of medicine and psychiatry is necessary to decide which interpretation is correct.

The acceptance of a sick role is implicit in every doctor–patient relationship. A person who seeks advice for health reasons (or for whom advice is sought by a third party) is at least temporarily in a dependent position. Something is recognized to be wrong and in need of putting right, and all workers in the caring professions, be they doctors, nurses, social workers, psychologists or occupational therapists, by offering any form of treatment are placing the patient in the sick role. Where the integrated model diverges from the disease model is in still giving responsibility to the patient for a substantial part of treatment. The patient is not merely a passive recipient of therapy but an active participant, to a lesser degree in stage five than stage one, but always having some active role.

The part of the psychodynamic model that applies throughout all phases of the hierarchical model is the awareness that the problems patients present to the doctor are only the tip of the iceberg. There are many unconscious, preconscious and conscious processes involved before the final form of the complaint is established, and this may be far removed from the underlying cause, as for example in the case of a hysterical symptom. Throughout assessment and treatment of a patient, the doctor has to be sensitive to other forms of communication and able to get across to the patient that he understands and is competent to deal with mental suffering. This quality is called empathy. The doctor also needs to be aware that the relationship he or she has with the patient can affect the outcome of therapy markedly, and by being sensitive to the nature of this relationship it can be used positively.

The behavioural model reminds us that what we too can determine our subsequent behaviour. 'Habit is the flywheel of society', wrote William James, and when habits are healthy all goes well. When they become maladaptive they unfortunately tend to reinforce the maladaptation, and behavioural techniques are needed to modify them. Most of this does not pass under the form of specialized therapy. For example, the upbringing of almost all children involves reward for doing what is thought to be good and praiseworthy, and punishment for what is thought to be wrong. In pathological states there is apparent punishment for good and reward for bad behaviour. Unsuccessful suicide develops positive reinforcement from the subsequent attention, and if this is not recognized the cycle may be perpetuated until eventually the patient actually does commit suicide, by mistake. Providing we balance the needs of patient and society the behavioural approach can be relevant at all stages of illness.

Cognition is part of living. The ability to react intelligently and rationally to changing circumstances separates man from all other species. During the course of mental illness thinking can get stuck in tramlines and the job of cognitive therapy is to release it from these fixed courses.

The aspect of the social model that runs throughout the correlative model is the aetiological one. Many forms of psychiatric illness can be the result of social forces acting on vulnerable individuals. No patient can be studied in isolation and an awareness of social and cultural background is necessary to understand both the nature and form of psychiatric disorder. An increasingly important part of mental disorder is transcultural psychiatry, which recognizes that although psychiatric illness may be fundamentally the same the world over, the relative frequency of disorder varies greatly from culture to culture, and the form that the illness takes even more so. Significantly altering social factors is difficult and again the needs of the individual have to be balanced against those of society. In major social reorganization such as planning a new town, the preventive importance of good planning in maintaining health deserves particular attention.

The doctor needs to incorporate all these points from our five previous models into the integrated hierarchical one. At initial assessment of the patient he will concentrate on getting enough information to summarize the problem formally. This will comprise factual, historical material derived from following the procedure given earlier in the account of the disease model (the data base) with corroboration of this where necessary from an independent informant, and an examination of the physical and mental state. The interview will also be used to build up a trusting relationship with the patient so that it does not consist of a series of brutal questions and answers but a gentle exploration of the problem. Even if the patient is apparently out of touch with his surroundings, whether or not he is suffering from a psychotic illness, the interview should proceed in the same gentle manner so that the foundations of mutual respect can be established. This may sound odd to those who have had to deal with violent people who are obviously 'mad' in the lay sense and psychotic in the medical one, but such patients can still appreciate good manners and careful handling although at the time they may not show it. The first interview usually sets the seal on the relationship at subsequent interviews and if it is handled badly the lost ground may never be recovered.

Once a diagnostic formulation and the level of illness has been established a plan of management is determined. This will depend on the nature and level of the illness and may consist of more than one approach for conditions that show elements of two levels. To a greater or lesser degree, depending on the state of the disorder, this plan will be discussed with the patient and approval sought. Approval may not always be given for conditions at level five of the model but the treatment may nevertheless have to be given compulsorily. In most instances approval for the passive component of treatment is readily given by the patient, for after all, they make no contribution towards it. More difficulty may be reached in agreeing on the active component and it may take some time before this is properly established. This does not prevent the passive form of treatment going ahead but it should be discussed as soon as possible once a plan of management has been decided. It is fairly easy to treat a patient with a chronic drinking problem initially as the first stage is to withdraw the alcohol under supervision but the patient's participation is so much more important in the later phases.

As treatment progresses the patient will pass down the hierarchy of the integrated model. There should be no difficulty in the therapist accommodating to this change in levels. He has already

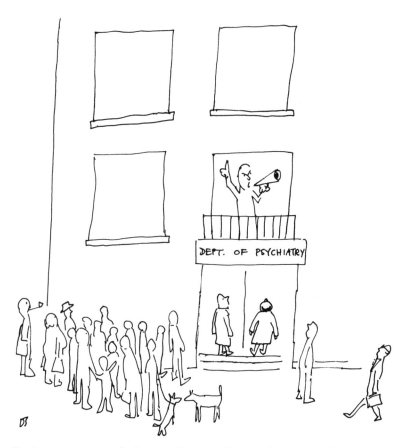

'It is not part of the professional's work to produce social
reform . . .'

established the different levels of treatment with the patient and so
does not give the impression of inconsistency or radical change of
mind. The relationship between therapist and patient becomes more
important in the cognitive, behavioural and psychodynamic stages
of the model and is one reason for maintaining continuity of care in
these stages. Major disruption can result if the patient is confronted
by a different therapist at each succeeding level and establishing a
relationship has to begin all over again. However, when the patient
has reached the social level of illness some boundary would have to
be drawn between the responsibility of mental heatlh professionals
and that of the wider community. It is not part of the professional's

emergence of the fourth stage. Attempts to adjust to the loss appear to cease altogether and other people are unable to alter her move towards isolation. Finally she develops a depressive psychosis, with delusions of poverty, unworthiness and guilt, accompanied by paranoid ideas and auditory hallucinations of an unpleasant critical kind. These tell her she is useless and that suuicide is the only way out of the burden she is causing to her friends and relatives. At this stage she no longer feels ill but wicked. The characteristic bodily changes of severe depression, including marked loss of weight and appetite, constipation, sleep disturbance with waking in the early hours, and a worsening of her depressed mood with feelings of complete hopelessness and worthlessness are present. As she feels such a burden on everyone and with such low self-esteem it is not surprising that she now contemplates suicide. Meanwhile, she elicits a range of reactions from other people: sympathy, anxiety, sadness, anger and mixed feelings too.

Other disorders may only show obvious evidence of one of these phases, others two or three, but in all instances there is the possibility that the disorder can present at any of the five levels. How can this be explained?

Hierarchy of Models

We are all aware of hierarchies in our lives. We all have to deal with much larger amounts of information than our brains can cope with and we order these in a way that leads to greatest efficiency. In addition to our own internal hierarchies we have external ones, most obvious in the structures of large organizations. Typically the bottom level of the organization contains the most people and the top level the least. A general feature of a hierarchy is that those on higher levels incorporate the characteristics of the lower levels. Thus the chairman of a large international company is regarded as representing the company at all levels. Thus, for example, if there is a major scandal involving a functioning of the lowest level of the organization the chairman may be regarded as responsible and forced to resign even though he had no direct knowledge of the circumstances and personnel involved in the scandal.

Models in psychiatry have a similar hierarchical structure and this is shown in Figure 7.2. The most minor mental illness (e.g. feeling angry and upset after failing a job interview) does not qualify for any diagnostic label but certainly creates social dysfunction and involves the social model. However, when specific symptoms are established at the second level of the hierarchy the psychodynamic

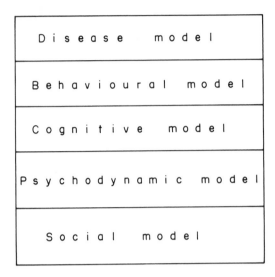

Fig 7.2   A hierarchy of models. Note that this is a true hierarchy in which each higher level comprises its own level and the features of all lower levels

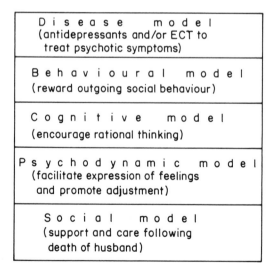

Fig 7.3   Matching models with treatment in Mrs X

model may be used. When maladaptive thinking predominates, the cognitive model is most appropriate and if the abnormality shows mainly in behaviour, the behavioural model applies. The hierarchy leads directly to an appropriate programme of treatment, which can incorporate treatment from the same level as the model together with treatment beneath it (Figure 7.3).

Matching Levels and Models

It will not have escaped attention that the models of mental disorder discussed in earlier chapters match these levels of illness in many respects. The hierarchical model states that for each stage of psychiatric disorder there is an aprpopriate model but the application of that model is only correct for that level of disorder. When the disorder moves to a different level, another model (or models) should be used. The level of disorder corresponds with the model used. This model could be identified as the medical model, in the sense that medical is a comprehensive term used to describe all aspects of caring. As pointed out, this term has been interpreted in many quarters as the disease model and for this reason we prefer the description as the hierarchical model.

At the first level of illness, which only comprizes minor changes of the level of feelings, formal psychiatric attention is rarely needed, and the social model is appropriate. When specific symptoms are established in the second level the pschodynamic model may be used. When maladaptive behaviour-responses are present in the third level, the behavioural model applies, and when irrational thinking is dominant in the fourth level the cognitive model applies: The disease model should be reserved for the severe manifestations of the fifth level. Because the different levels can all be shown at different times in the course of an illness the therapist cannot presume that any one model is suitable for a particular disorder. Nevertheless, because some disorders predominantly are expressed at one level there will be a tendency for one model to predominate.

In our introduction we emphasized that models are only of use if they fit the facts closely and provide a coherent basis for intervention. They are practical instruments rather than theoretical abstractions. To test whether this particular combination of models has any value we need to see whether our new correlative model is consistent with good psychiatric practice and whether it has any predictive value.

Fifth level—disease model To return to our depressed patient, does our model help us to understand and treat her problem (Figure 7.3).

Most psychiatrists would see this patient at the fifth level, when her psychotic symptoms are established and admisson to hospital is often necessary because of the danger of successful suicide. It does not require a great deal of skill and intellect to appreciate that the depressive illness is in some way due the bereavement, but at this stage the underlying cause is not of immediate concern. The doctor is faced with a woman who is a suicidal risk, and possibly at risk of physical ill health because of poor nutrition and inadequate self-care. The patient is firmly placed in the sick role because she is sick. Her mental function is unbalanced because of the severity of this stage and decisions about treatment will have to be made independently and not necessarily with the patient's co-operation. Admission to hospital and treatment with ECT and antidepressant drugs may therefore have to be given without her permission. During this disease phase of treatment the hospital setting and attitudes of other patients, medical and nursing staff are largely immaterial, although they will become very important as recovery progresses and should not be ignored now.

Fourth level—cognitive model As the patient's psychotic symptoms improve, the negative thinking behind the depression will become more prominent. Feelings of guilt, blaming herself for her husband's death and believing that she cannot live without him, are inappropriate assumptions that will prolong the depression. The depression must be prevented from returning to its former cognitive 'set' in which all possibility of improvement is excluded and morbid thinking preoccupies her brain. At a fairly simple level, and certainly one which has not required the skills of a cognitive therapist, staff on the ward can explore the patient's feelings and beliefs in a gentle way that helps her to understand that she can adjust to the death of her husband without being a traitor to his memory.

Third level—behavioural model As the patient responds to treatment she will lose her delusions and hallucinations but remain socially withdrawn. She will probably be reluctant to eat regularly and wish to spend most of her time alone. During this time there is a danger that ruminating about her husband will again lead to a return of severe depressive symptoms. The nursing staff react to this withdrawal with a form of operant conditioning. They will positively reinforce socially outgoing behaviour but will be careful not to negatively reinforce the withdrawal by any form of punishment as they know that this can only reinforce the depression. They will encourage her to eat with other patients, talk to her socially instead of merely formally discussing her symptoms, and praise her when

she achieves small advances such as baking cakes for other patients in the occupational therapy department or takes part in group activities on the ward.

Second level—psychodynamic model As she improves in confidence and can face society again she will move towards the second level. This is the time to explore her thoughts and feelings about her dead husband, knowing that at first this may be a painful process. By 'working through' her loss again she can undergo the normal grieving process and restructure her world in a satisfactory and healthy way. It is likely that this stage could be carried out at a day hospital or in an outpatient clinic after discharge from in-patient care.

First level—social model The first level of disorder would predominate sometime later when she is probably attending as an outpatient to monitor progress. Although she has adjusted in many ways to the loss of her husband she cannot help being reminded of him as she sits in the house where they have spent so many years together. Provided that the treatment at the other four levels has been completed satisfactorily a change of accommodation, preferably to one where she has greater social contacts, is all that is necessary to complete the adjustment and treatment of her depressive illness.

When changing from one approach to another during the course of a disorder one is merely moving to a different level in the hierarchy (Figure 7.3). This is hardly a revolutionary concept but is rarely formalized. In general medicine a condition such as hypertension can be viewed similarly. At level five the important aspect is to bring the blood pressure down by drug therapy or similar medical means, but once this has been achieved the patient needs to have his individual needs and personality considered, and advice given about his lifestyle, occupational pressures and personal relationships, much of which may need to come from non-medical sources.

The hierarchical approach should also predict successfully that when the level of the disorder does not correspond then the approach will be unsuccessful. There is a popular, but now outmoded, view of schizophrenia that it is not a true illness but a natural reaction of man to the oppressive conformity of our society. The victim can only break out of the mould cast for him by society by apparently becoming mad in the form of schizophrenia. This serves as a vehicle to 'break through to health' and therefore, according to the hypothesis, it is best to treat the condition at the first stage of our model by altering society rather than the patient. When this theory

has been put to the test the evidence is universally negative. Patients do not achieve health by passing through a schizophrenic illness. If the condition is not treated using the disease model it is likely to become persistent, chronic and damage the personality irreparably. There is similar negative evidence that disorders in the first stage of illness can be treated by the disease stage of our model. It is of no value to treat people distressed and disadvantaged by poverty and poor housing by hospital admission and drug treatment. These changes will temporarily remove the unpleasant feelings but will not alter the underlying difficulties, and by 'medicalizing' the problem the patient may be prevented from taking action himself to change matters.

The demarcation lines are not so clearly drawn when intermediate phases are considered. For example, a severely agoraphobic patient who generally avoids all situations outside the home may be treated according to level three along behavioural lines. Gradual exposure to the feared situation or prevention of conditioned avoidance by remaining in the feared situation until anxiety is resolved may be successful but sometimes fails because of continued anxiety and panic. In the worst form of the disorder the patient has a 'pan-phobia' of everything and can be said to reach the fifth stage of the model. It is therefore appropriate to give drug treatment to reduce or suppress the panic feelings that are interfering with behaviour therapy. Similarly, a phobic patient who is responding to behaviour therapy may need cognitive therapy to prevent him from developing any new symptoms of anxiety by further phobic avoidance, and he may also need psychotherapeutic intervention to illustrate how the disorder has been manipulated (not necessarily consciously) by either the patient or close relatives for a variety of reasons. Unless this is resolved the phobias may return.

Cause and Pathology

It is possible to match the causes of mental disorder with levels in a similar way to that for treatment, but care is needed in defining cause, or to use its more technical synonym, aetiology. Just as an illness can manifest features of all five levels at different times so can its cause affect all five levels. A distinction is often made between 'causes' and 'triggering events' but this defines the level rather than a fundamental difference. Triggering events are usually at level one in the hierarchical model but they can lead to changes at other levels, and the nature of the disorder is the resultant of all these changes.

It is wrong to define any mental disorder by its apparent cause because of variability in response. Thus the term 'reactive depression' should be discarded because it implies a different type of depression than, for example, so-called 'endogenous depression'. If the 'reaction', whatever its nature, leads to significant deficiency in brain levels of certain amines (5-hydroxy-tryptamine and noradrenaline), then the clinical presentation will be the same as that for the (apparently) endogenously-depressed patient. The reaction has taken place at level one but led to changes at level five, and these determine the nature of the depression.

Most mental disorders are reactive in one sense, in that their timing is determined by one or more external precipitants.

Underlying predisposition, however, really decides the nature of the disorder and it is this level of aetiology that correlates with presentation of illness. Let us take an example to illustrate the importance of underlying predisposition in determining mental illness and how it is linked to aetiology.

Five people, who we shall call A, B, C, D and E, are involved in a road traffic accident but not seriously injured. Subject A is of stable personality and has never had any mental illness. She recovers rapidly from the experience but for a short period prefers to travel by train rather than by car when she has a choice. Subject B is a somewhat insecure anxiety-prone man who has never adjusted to leaving his mother six years previously. He becomes much more anxious after the accident and has acute episodes of panic for no apparent reason. Subject C has a mother who has suffered from agoraphobia when she was a child. She has never had agoraphobia before but after the accident she developed some phobia of car travel. This later generalizes to all travelling outside the house so that she becomes severely agoraphobic. Subject D becomes depressed after the accident and cannot stop ruminating about death and his own mortality. Subject E has a father and grandfather who have had episodes of severe depression and he too has previously been in hospital with episodes of depression and hypomania. He appears not to react to the accident at first but a few weeks later he suddenly becomes overactive and restless, needing little sleep, shows elation and irritability alternately, and plans to build a space ship to take him to Mars as the prospect of continued life on Earth is not exciting.

All these five people have been through the same experience but react differently because of different combinations of aetiological factors. Subject A reacts only to the accident, which can be said to be as much related to social forces as vehicular ones (level one). Subject B reactivates unresolved anxiety that stems from his relationship

with his mother (level two). Subject C becomes agoraphobic which generalized avoidance, a pattern of behaviour she has developed at least as much from modelling herself on her agoraphobic mother as a child as on genetic predisposition (level three). Subject D develops persistent depressive thinking. Subject E enters a manic phase (level five) of his manic-depressive illness for which the accident may be seen as an important, though non-specific triggering event. But of course all five (level four) individuals have been through the same experience and so the aetiological factors of the first level are relevant to a varying degree in their resulting problems. Allowing room for simultaneous aetiological factors from different levels removes much of othe controversy about the correct way to regard psychiatric illness. Although a condition may be triggered by social factors that is no reason to regard social forms of management as the only appropriate ones; it is the end result to the triggering that determines the best line of treatment.

Both types of pathology are similarly explained by using the hierarchy. Pathology not only means gross changes in bodily organs such as the loss of brain cells and flattening of the grooves (sulci) in the brain in conditions such as senile dementia; it describes abnormalities at other levels also. So in psychoses well-known phrases such as 'ideas of reference' and 'delusional perception' are examples of descriptive psychopathology, and the maladaptive behaviour patterns of stage three, the dynamic psychopathology of stage two, and the social pathology of stage one are all manifestations of the form of illness. As long as one level of pathology is not applied to an inappropriate stage—for example it would be nonsense to describe someone in a depressive stupor as displaying introjection and repression—then there is no difficulty in fitting pathology to the model.

Prevention

Prevention also follows the multimodel pattern of aetiology. It is appropriate for any preventive measure to be given provided that it matches the mental disorder at one level at least. Thus patients with recurrent episodes of mania and depression may take the treatment from stage five of our model, the drug lithium carbonate, even when they are completely well and outside the scope of our model altogether. But it would be inappropriate to give antidepressant tablets to a population living in squalid stressful conditions on the grounds that it would prevent them from becoming depressed.

How do we go about using the hierarchical approach in practice? First of all there are some parts of each of the models described previously that can be incorporated into our model as general rules. The two aspects of the disease model that apply to all levels of illness are the need for a formalized assessment of every mental problem and the acceptance that in a doctor–patient relationship the patient has to adopt a sick role at some stage, even if it is only at the beginning. The need for a formalized assessment will already be obvious to the reader. This assessment would be usually made at a first interview and involves a judicious mix of direct questions from the interviewer and spontaneous description of problems by the patient. A proper history of the problem and an assessment of the current mental state of the patient are essential parts, for without them much relevant material will remain undetected. The interviewer's assessment will be summarized in a formulation of the problem in aetiological, diagnostic and prognostic terms.

We should also like the doctor to describe which stage of the illness the patient has reached as this will influence management, but as he will look in vain for any indication of this in psychiatric text books we shall have to ask him to use his own judgement in deciding this question. This judgement will require both an objective assessment of the patient's state and a recording of the patient's own views about his attitudes and feelings towards his problem. Sometimes these will vary; the patient may think his attacks of sweating and palpitations signify organic disease whereas the doctor will view them as anxiety symptoms. A sound knowledge of medicine and psychiatry is necessary to decide which interpretation is correct.

The acceptance of a sick role is implicit in every doctor–patient relationship. A person who seeks advice for health reasons (or for whom advice is sought by a third party) is at least temporarily in a dependent position. Something is recognized to be wrong and in need of putting right, and all workers in the caring professions, be they doctors, nurses, social workers, psychologists or occupational therapists, by offering any form of treatment are placing the patient in the sick role. Where the integrated model diverges from the disease model is in still giving responsibility to the patient for a substantial part of treatment. The patient is not merely a passive recipient of therapy but an active participant, to a lesser degree in stage five than stage one, but always having some active role.

The part of the psychodynamic model that applies throughout all phases of the hiearchical model is the awareness that the problems patients present to the doctor are only the tip of the iceberg. There are many unconscious, preconscious and conscious processes

involved before the final form of the complaint is established, and this may be far removed from the underlying cause, as for example in the case of a hysterical symptom. Throughout assessment and treatment of a patient, the doctor has to be sensitive to other forms of communication and able to get across to the patient that he understands and is competent to deal with mental suffering. This quality is called empathy. The doctor also needs to be aware that the relationship he or she has with the patient can affect the outcome of therapy markedly, and by being sensitive to the nature of this relationship it can be used positively.

The behavioural model reminds us that what we too can determine our subsequent behaviour. 'Habit is the flywheel of society', wrote William James, and when habits are healthy all goes well. When they become maladaptive they unfortunately tend to reinforce the maladaptation, and behavioural techniques are needed to modify them. Most of this does not pass under the form of specialized therapy. For example, the upbringing of almost all children involves reward for doing what is thought to be good and praiseworthy, and punishment for what is thought to be wrong. In pathological states there is apparent punishment for good and reward for bad behaviour. Unsuccessful suicide develops positive reinforcement from the subsequent attention, and if this is not recognized the cycle may be perpetuated until eventually the patient actually does commit suicide, by mistake. Providing we balance the needs of patient and society the behavioural approach can be relevant at all stages of illness.

Cognition is part of living. The ability to react intelligently and rationally to changing circumstances separates man from all other species. During the course of mental illness thinking can get stuck in tramlines and the job of cognitive therapy is to release it from these fixed courses.

The aspect of the social model that runs throughout the correlative model is the aetiological one. Many forms of psychiatric illness can be the result of social forces acting on vulnerable individuals. No patient can be studied in isolation and an awareness of social and cultural background is necessary to understand both the nature and form of psychiatric disorder. An increasingly important part of mental disorder is transcultural psychiatry, which recognizes that although psychiatric illness may be fundamentally the same the world over, the relative frequency of disorder varies greatly from culture to culture, and the form that the illness takes even more so. Significantly altering social factors is difficult and again the needs of the individual have to be balanced against those of society. In major social reorganization such as planning a new town, the preventive

importance of good planning in maintaining health deserves particular attention.

The doctor needs to incorporate all these points from our five previous models into the integrated hierarchical one. At initial assessment of the patient he will concentrate on getting enough information to summarize the problem formally. This will comprise factual, historical material derived from following the procedure given earlier in the account of the disease model (the data base) with corroboration of this where necessary from an independent informant, and an examination of the physical and mental state. The interview will also be used to build up a trusting relationship with the patient so that it does not consist of a series of brutal questions and answers but a gentle exploration of the problem. Even if the patient is apparently out of touch with his surroundings, whether or not he is suffering from a psychotic illness, the interview should proceed in the same gentle manner so that the foundations of mutual respect can be established. This may sound odd to those who have had to deal with violent people who are obviously 'mad' in the lay sense and psychotic in the medical one, but such patients can still appreciate good manners and careful handling although at the time they may not show it. The first interview usually sets the seal on the relationship at subsequent interviews and if it is handled badly the lost ground may never be recovered.

Once a diagnostic formulation and the level of illness has been established a plan of management is determined. This will depend on the nature and level of the illness and may consist of more than one approach for conditions that show elements of two levels. To a greater or lesser degree, depending on the state of the disorder, this plan will be discussed with the patient and approval sought. Approval may not always be given for conditions at level five of the model but the treatment may nevertheless have to be given compulsorily. In most instances approval for the passive component of treatment is readily given by the patient, for after all, they make no contribution towards it. More difficulty may be reached in agreeing on the active component and it may take some time before this is properly established. This does not prevent the passive form of treatment going ahead but it should be discussed as soon as possible once a plan of management has been decided. It is fairly easy to treat a patient with a chronic drinking problem initially as the first stage is to withdraw the alcohol under supervision but the patient's participation is so much more important in the later phases.

As treatment progresses the patient will pass down the hierarchy of the integrated model. There should be no difficulty in the therapist accommodating to this change in levels. He has already

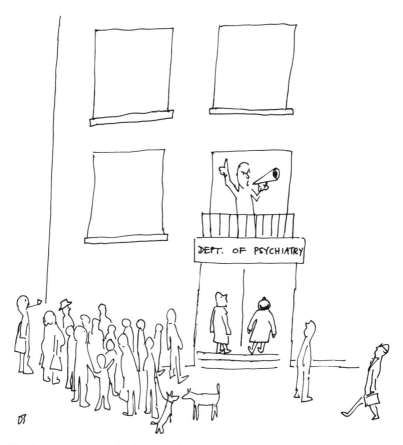

'It is not part of the professional's work to produce social reform . . .'

established the different levels of treatment with the patient and so does not give the impression of inconsistency or radical change of mind. The relationship between therapist and patient becomes more important in the cognitive, behavioural and psychodynamic stages of the model and is one reason for maintaining continuity of care in these stages. Major disruption can result if the patient is confronted by a different therapist at each succeeding level and establishing a relationship has to begin all over again. However, when the patient has reached the social level of illness some boundary would have to be drawn between the responsibility of mental heatlh professionals and that of the wider community. It is not part of the professional's

work to produce social reform, although many take up this issue independently of their mental health role. Psychiatrists in particular have sometimes overstretched their boundaries and incorporated their models into the whole framework of society. This is not wise.

Once the importance of looking at different stages of illness in different ways is appreciated, much of the bitter argument within the psychiatric profession and between other professionals disappears. The integrated approach does not mean a patient should be treated in the same way at all times, and dogmatic adherence to one particular model is a source of much conflict. Much depends on the training of professionals and who they see in their working lives. Social workers (apart from specialist mental health ones) see many of their clients at level one, psychoanalysts and psychotherapists treat their patients at level two, clinical psychologists practise their skills derived from learning theory under cognitive model at levels three and four, and hospital-orientated psychiatrists see patients predominantly at the fifth level. This leads to a blinkered view of psychiatric existence. The social worker is often shocked when he or she hears of a client known for years to have major social difficulties is in a mental hospital and has been treated with ECT. This is an understandable response as the social worker's experience with the client has been almost entirely of the lower levels of the hierarchy. We all have the capacity to become psychotically ill and to require treatment at the disease level of the hierarchy. As one past president of the Royal College of Psychiatrists has put it, 'every citizen should have the right to be admitted against his or her will, to be treated without loss of dignity, in a first class psychiatric service' (Birley 1991).

The patient with psychotic depression in hospital is very different from the one with problems at home seen by the social worker. Of course they are the same person but the condition is as different from the ill person with pneumonia who is out of breath compared with his healthy self when he is breathless after running for a bus. If mental health professionals were able to see psychiatric patients at all levels of the model there would be much more understanding and less sniping at other's points of view.

All parts of the integrated model can link together harmoniously provided that it is clear which part is operative at any one time. This decision is not a fixed one, as advances in knowledge are always taking place that change our concepts of mental disorder. If, for example, it is confirmed that schizophrenia is an organic disease with structural changes in the brain, it becomes much more appropriate to treat most of its manifestations according to stage five. The other four stages of the model still have a place once the major abnormality has been treated. There is also a major challenge for the model in the assessment and management of personality disorder. These conditions describe persistent maladaptive aspects of personality functioning that lead to impaired social function and influence the outcome of many mental illnesses. Personality disorders represent a challenge to the integrated model because it asks all parts of the model to work in unison.

We are not pretending that the integrated model is going to solve all the difficulties of divergent schools in psychiatry. But we look on it as a good working hypothesis that should aid clinical practice. It should also give a theoretical base to the eclectic approach to psychiatry. The original eclectics were members of a school of Greek philosophy who had no doctrines of their own but borrowed ideas from other schools whenever it suited them. Not surprisingly they were not thought of very highly, and were considered to be third-rate philosophers who did not have sufficient originality to develop ideas of their own. The same image has tended to follow psychiatrists who regard themselves as eclectic. It may seem reasonable to choose the approach that best suits the situation but if this is just a personal decision it lacks any general application and its practitioners are just dilettantes. We hope that the integrated model can be viewed as an eclectic's charter, giving a basis for good practice in psychiatry which can be developed and taught to others instead of accruing only from prolonged clinical experience.

TEAMWORK WITH THE INTEGRATED MODEL

It will be quickly appreciated by the reader that good psychiatry must involve close team working if all five models are to be integrated. This is not easy. There has to be recognition of the many different ways in which psychiatric disorders can present to professionals (and non-professionals) and that these can change over time.

This is most marked in the area of child and adolescent psychiatry, where developmental and interactional factors combine. This is to be expected in a field which deals with babies at one extreme and young adults at the other. Young people develop and undergo an extraordinary degree of change as they grow—physically, intellectually, in terms of the acquisition of skills and behaviour (e.g. reading, social skills) and in terms of what is expected of them. To take only one obvious example, a 2-year-old baby will not toddle along to a doctor complaining of depression; a 17-year-old might; and a 12-year-old might or might not, and more likely would be taken by his or her parents, they perhaps more concerned about the child's symptoms than is the boy or girl. The presentation and nature of disorders in childhood and adolescence change too, so that what we think of as 'depression' might manifest as feeding problems in an infant, misbehaviour and school problems in middle childhood, and adult-type depressive symptoms in adolescence.

Thus things change as development proceeds: the child changes, the presentation of disorder changes, and quite probably at least some of the mechanisms underlying disorder change too. Childhood disorder is therefore conceptualized in *developmental* terms, rather than in the relatively stable concepts of adult psychiatry where changes in personality, disorder and circumstances can be less dramatic.

Secondly, these changing internal and external influences and processes *interact* in a complicated way. Clarifying this requires information drawn from many different fields, including many different aspects of social, biological and psychological science; Rutter (1980) provides an excellent review of the field. In so far as the approach can be summed up in a sentence or two, it is based on the recognition that as development proceeds various inherent characteristics emerge and mature, and various external influences interact with these characteristics, which may then become modified. However, these modified characteristics in turn influence *other* individual characteristics and the environment, and both of the latter may change too. This model, then, is one of a constant spiralling of complex interactions within the individual and between the individual and the external world.

To take a simple example: a poor single woman, a heavy smoker, has her child in a poor neighbourhood where obstetric and paediatric facilities are less than ideal. Her low self-esteem and general level of expectations means that she does not use the reasonable antenatal advice and care that is available, and she does not complain about poor service from doctors and nurses. Her own family background has taught her to be compliant. The baby is born somewhat underweight and rather hard to manage: slow to suckle, easily upset, slow to develop predictable habits. The vulnerable mother loses heart and gets irritable with the child, which makes matters worse for both. They upset each other, and in the next few years she is more or less constantly depressed, the child irritable, enuretic and overactive, the problems for which he is referred. He goes to a rough school in a rough neighbourhood, learns little and goes from bad to worse.

The 'advice' implied by this sketch, whether as health advice and education, as social policy, or as care in the individual case, clearly includes matters to do with basic physical health and care for mothers and babies; the upbringing of children; the psychology of motherhood; the quality and accessibility of obstetric and paediatric services; and to do with schooling. In addition, the child may or may not have a clinical disorder.

These complexities are organized in diagnostic assessment by using the multi-axial approach described earlier, in which factors are teased out in terms of individual disorder, if any, developmental delay, intellectual level, physical health and psychosocial circumstances. The formulation in child and adolescent psychiatry is made in similar terms.

Earlier, we described the process of assessment as consisting partly of *description* of the problem in ordinary language, and partly of *explanation* in which complex models are used. If we take this approach we will often be left with two sets of problems: problems which, once clarified, can be dealt with by (for example) a referred child's parents and teachers; and problems for which psychiatric help is more appropriate.

This is where teamwork comes in and where an integrated model shows its spurs. All psychiatrists, not just child and adolescent ones, have to work with a range of other professionals, those from inside and outside the mental health services, to meet the needs of referred patients. Team working characteristically involves joint assessment and allocation so that a key worker from an appropriate discipline takes on the main clinical responsibility. For example, if the child in the above example was referred to a psychiatrist, it could well turn out that the psychiatrist, an educational psychologist, schoolteachers and the local practice's health visitor would need to collaborate not only with each other but with the child's mother. This does not mean everyone working at once with mother and child, falling over each other in the process, but helping both school and mother to handle the child along sensible and consistent lines. In a case like this the psychiatrist may not need to do any clinical work with the referred child, but simply take an *advisory* or *consultative* role, perhaps with health visitor and school. Alternatively, he might work directly with the child, the mother, or both together; in which case he would be doing *family work*. This may consist of *family therapy*, using a systems-based or psychodynamic model, or he may help the mother use a *behavioural or cognitive* approach (Steinberg 1983, 1986; Steinberg & Yule 1985).

The concept of case or care management enshrines this notion of team working with appropriate levels of responsibility. Good team working requires the integrated model we have put forward if it is not to lead to sterile arguments between disciplines that serve only to fragment care. There are many ways of organizing good team working and case management (Onyett 1992) but all require a common base of knowledge and philosophy. The integrated hierarchical model of mental disorders offers this.

THE IMPORTANCE OF CONSULTATION

Consultative approaches are worth a little elaboration here. They do not of course constitute a model for mental disorder as such, but represent a way of standing back from the technical questions of diagnosis and treatment and posing a different set of questions, and moreover ones framed in ordinary language. For example: what's going on here? what's going right, and what's going wrong? who's involved, who cares, and who ought to be taking responsibility in the presenting situation? What's the best way of proceeding? Who should be doing what, for whom and with whom?

In many areas of general medicine, and much of psychiatry, there are already clear answers to such questions. Clinical practice is so well established with dealing with such questions in, for example, acute appendicitis, meningitis, epidemic diseases, fractures and so on, that the questions are hardly noticed. Many areas of general and particularly child psychiatry however generate issues that are less clear cut. Thus psychiatry may have a part to play in the management of, say, delinquency, stress at work, problems in schools, family difficulties and the emotional and psychosomatic problems that arise in the whole of the rest of medicine, but each situation is likely to be different. If every case that *might* need psychiatric care were to have the benefit of a comprehensive clinical work-up from a psychiatric team, there would not only never be time for treatment, but also there would never be the time or resources to respond to every request for an assessment. A little time ago the distinguished psychiatrist Norman Sartorius was asked what he considered to be the most important psychiatric discovery of the past 50 years. To the surprise of many people he cited the observation that most psychiatric disorder throughout the world was seen and managed not by psychiatrists but by those in primary care. This indeed is the issue, or at least part of it, and in the consultative model we have a practical way of responding, not by a full-blown clinical intervention, but from a rather wider perspective that does not assume that clinical intervention will be needed.

The essence of the consultative approach is that the technical expert (in this case, the psychiatrist) does not 'take over', but tries to help the front-line worker who is making the referral. Thus a teacher can be helped to manage a difficult pupil, or a residential social worker helped with a group of disturbed children, without the young people concerned having to be booked into the local clinic for a full-scale history-taking and examination. Similarly a paediatrician or a general practitioner may welcome consultation of this sort as an alternative to a straight referral, in some cases.

When one professional worker helps another in this way, instead of simply taking the case on in the more traditional manner, both learn from the experience, and the worker accepting this sort of response may well find his or her skills in managing future similar cases enhanced. The consultative approach, therefore, not only makes sense where referrals to specialist services may be arbitrary, but has an educational component too. It also generates questions which may be at the same time both naive and valuable; for example, in a school or children's home, *why* does the teacher or social worker not have the time, energy or encouragement to apply their basic skills to a child's problem? What would it take for them to be able to do so? And so on. The consultative model of care is therefore different from the clinical model, and may be an alternative to it, or a supplement; thus the psychiatrist and teacher may negotiate that the psychiatrist will deal with one agreed part of the problem and the teacher with the rest.

Consultation in this sense is a development of the past 20 years or so, simple in its principles and quite radical in some of its implications. It is a technique that incoporates joint problem-clarifying and problem-solving strategies, and it teaches and generates questions as it goes. It might even reduce waiting lists, or at least change the nature of the problems in the queues to see the psychiatrist. This is not the place to describe this work in detail but its scope is discussed elsewhere (Steinberg 1989, 1992a, 1992b).

CONCLUSION

We have seen that quite different conceptual models can be used, separately or together, to help make sense of the problems with which psychiatrists are presented, to understand mental dysfunction, and to plan preventive work, management strategies and specific approaches to treatment. They also help us frame hypotheses for research purposes. In clinical or academic practice, the willingness to acknowledge the contribution of quite different models leads to important findings; the recent research linking structural brain change, response to drugs and the importance of family dynamics in schizophrenia, is only one example. A growing number of similar examples may be found in modern textbooks of psychiatry. It may be that in the future, remarkable specific discoveries will be made, equivalent to the discovery at the turn of the century that the syphilitic spirochaete caused general paralysis of the insane, the psychiatric complication of syphilis. But in our present state of understanding, nearly a century later, the skilled use of refined conceptual models in combination seems to offer the most hope for useful work and further progress in treatment and prevention.

Our advice to the serious student is to keep an open mind about the helpfulness, in clinical practice, of the different models, and not to be seduced by the superficial attractiveness of one, however well presented. Variety is the stuff of psychiatry and those who imprison

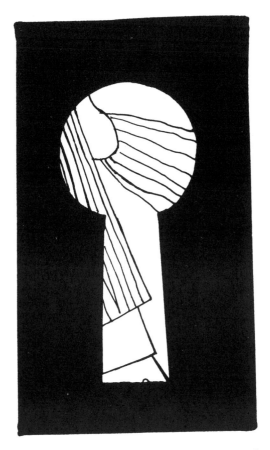

'. . . those who imprison themselves within the confines of one model have only the perspective of the keyhole . . .'

themselves within the confines of one model only have the perspective of the keyhole, a perspective that is stimulating at first but without wider involvement will end up as seriously limiting. Good models are vehicles to progress, and although we may develop a sentimental attachment to one, it will need to be replaced when it starts breaking down.

REFERENCES

American Psychiatric Association (1980) *Diagnostic and Statistical Manual for Mental Disorders, 3rd revision.* American Psychiatric Association, Washington.

Birley, J.L.T. (1991) Psychiatrists and citizens. *British Journal of Psychiatry,* **159**, 1–6.

Foucault, M. (1967) *Madness and Civilisation.* Tavistock, London.

Lewis, A. (1953) Health as a social concept. *British Journal of Sociology,* **4**, 109–124.

Onyett, S. (1992) *Case Management in Mental Health.* Chapman and Hall, London.

Ramon, S. (1985) *Psychiatry in Britain: Meaning and Policy.* Croom Helm, London.

Rutter, M. (1980) (ed) *Developmental Psychiatry.* Heinemann, London.

Steinberg, D. (1983) *The Clinical Psychiatry of Adolescence, Clinical Work from a Social and Developmental Perspective.* Wiley, Chichester.

Steinberg, D. (1986) (ed) *The Adolescent Unit: Work and Teamwork in Adolescent Psychiatry.* Wiley, Chichester.

Steinberg, D. (1989) *Interprofessional Consultation.* Blackwell Scientific Publications, Oxford.

Steinberg, D. (1992a) Consultative work in child and adolescent psychiatry. *Archives of Disease in Childhood,* **67**, 1302–1305.

Steinberg, D. (1992b) Psychiatry: concepts, principles and practicalities. In C.G.D. Brook (ed), *Adolescent Medicine,* Edward Arnold, Sevenoaks.

Steinberg, D. and Yule, W. (1985) *Consultative Work.* In M. Rutter and L. Hersov (eds) *Child and Adolescent Psychiatry: Modern Approaches.* Blackwell, Oxford.

Szasz, T.S. (1961) *The Myth of Mental Illness.* Harper and Row, New York.

World Helath Organisation (1992) *International Classification of Diseases,* 10th Edn. WHO, Geneva.

Index

Index compiled by Annette Musker